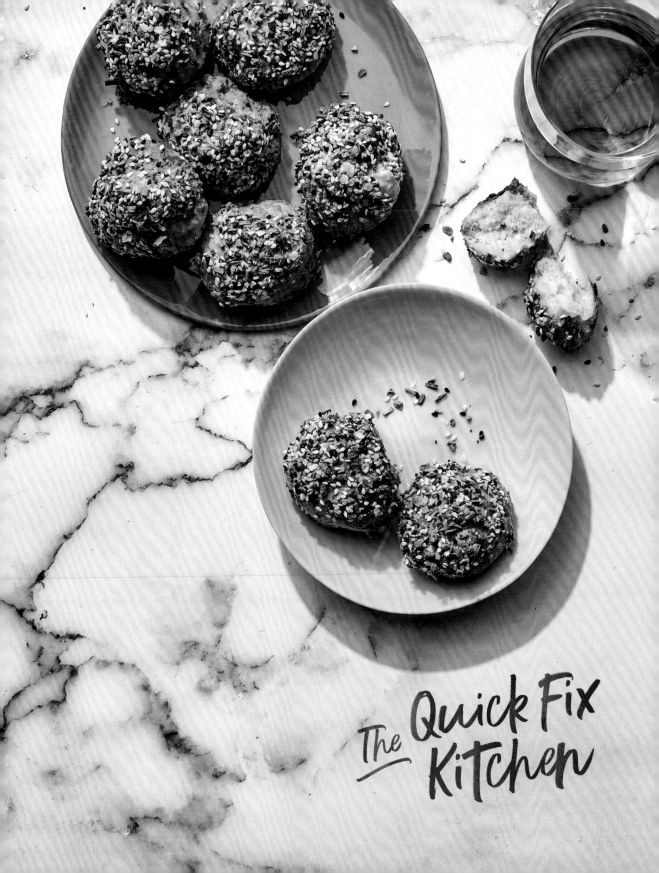

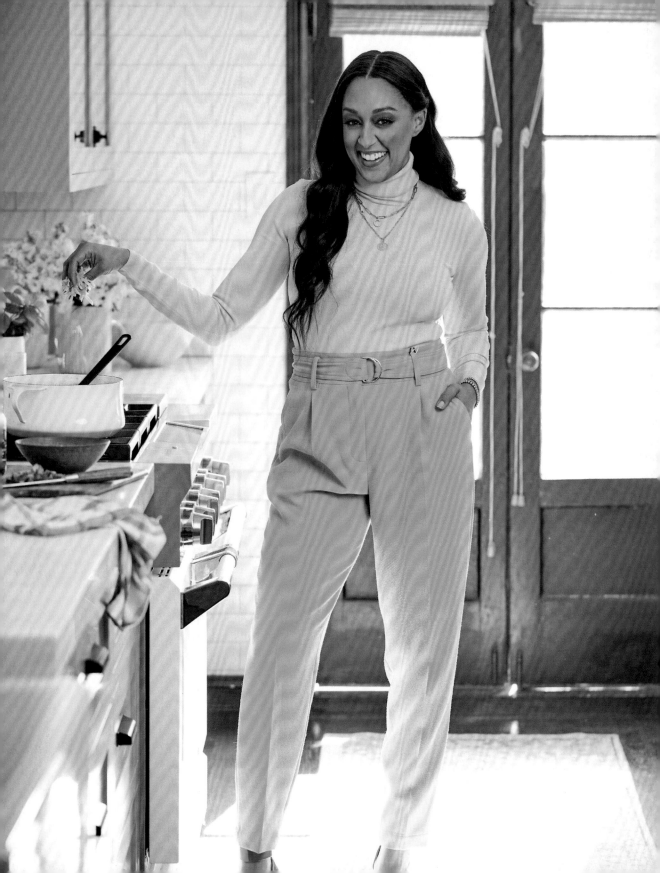

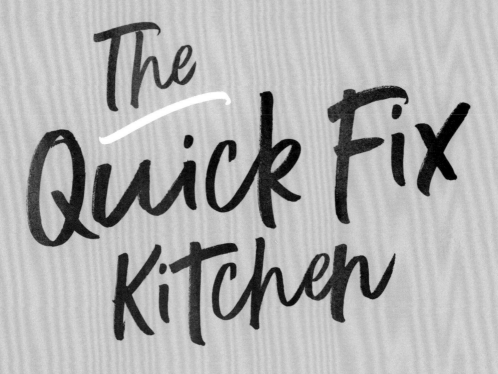

The Quick Fix Kitchen

EASY RECIPES & TIME-SAVING TIPS
FOR A HEALTHIER, STRESS-FREE LIFE

Tia Mowry

PHOTOGRAPHY BY MATT ARMENDARIZ

RODALE
NEW YORK

Copyright © 2021 by Tia Mowry-Hardrict
Photographs copyright © 2021 by Matt Armendariz

Published in the United States by Rodale Books,
an imprint of Random House, a division of
Penguin Random House LLC, New York.
rodalebooks.com

RODALE and the Plant colophon are registered
trademarks of Penguin Random House LLC.

Library of Congress Cataloging-in-Publication Data
Names: Mowry, Tia, author.
Title: The quick fix kitchen / by Tia Mowry.
Description: First edition.
     New York : Rodale Books, 2021.
     Includes bibliographical references
     and index. | Identifiers: LCCN 2020056470
     ISBN 9780593232828 (hardcover)
     ISBN 9780593232835 (ebook)
Subjects: LCSH: Quick and easy cooking.
     LCGFT: Cookbooks.
Classification: LCC TX833.5 .M69 2021
     DDC 641.5/12—dc23
LC record available at
     https://lccn.loc.gov/2020056470

ISBN 978-0-593-23282-8
Ebook ISBN 978-0-593-23283-5

Printed in China

Book and cover design by Chelsea Hunter

10 9 8 7 6 5 4 3 2 1

First Edition

I dedicate everything I do to my family. Nothing but gratitude for my best critics and taste testers: my husband, Cory, and our two kids, Cree and Cairo. You three are what keeps me motivated, focused, and joyful. Mommy loves you.

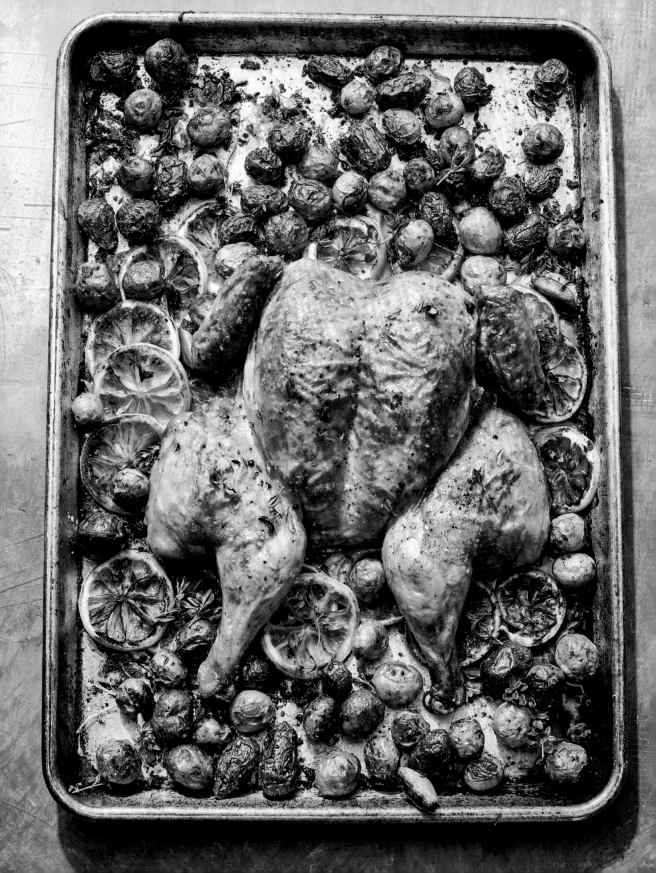

Contents

INTRODUCTION

tradition ⚬ noun

tra·di·tion |

\ trə-ˈdi-shən

the handing down of
information, beliefs, and
customs by word of mouth
or by example from one
generation to another
without written instruction

The road to this book is paved with a lifetime of family meals: from cooking as a household duty for my parents and siblings, to cooking as an absolute, always on my mind, hand me that apron and fire up the stove obsession. As a child, we didn't have the money to eat frequently at restaurants. Instead, my family gathered around our table at home, feasting on the meal one of us whipped up. It wasn't formal in any sense, but it gave us the opportunity to connect: no phones, no TV, just us and the nourishment on our plates. Our glass table, the Mowry symbol of togetherness, was the pillar of some of my fondest memories. Wherever my family moved, that table moved with us. And even though the dreaded task of cleaning it followed—spaghetti fingerprints and slurp splashes everywhere—it will forever remain close to my heart!

When I first started cooking, I assisted my mom by collecting ingredients and pushing a chair up to the counter to help. She guided me as I poured flour into the mixing bowl, cracked eggs into the pan (shells and all!), and tasted when she did. Whether or not it needed more salt or pepper, I had no clue. But when she asked for my opinion, I felt like an indispensable mini sous-chef, a magician's assistant helping conjure something from nothing. Eventually, cooking became a part of the chore cycle, and I took control of all the big-girl responsibilities: from seasoning the meat and chopping the carrots, celery, onions, and collards to setting the meal onto the table, lifting the lid from the pot, and watching the steam ascend.

At a young age, the obligation to cook for my family gave me structure, drove a new type of creativity, and built my confidence and humility. Mom's a drill sergeant, and when she told me to do something, you better believe I did it without a second thought! I learned through that experience, and through the mistakes I made. And you know, that's why I'm such a good cook today. Presenting

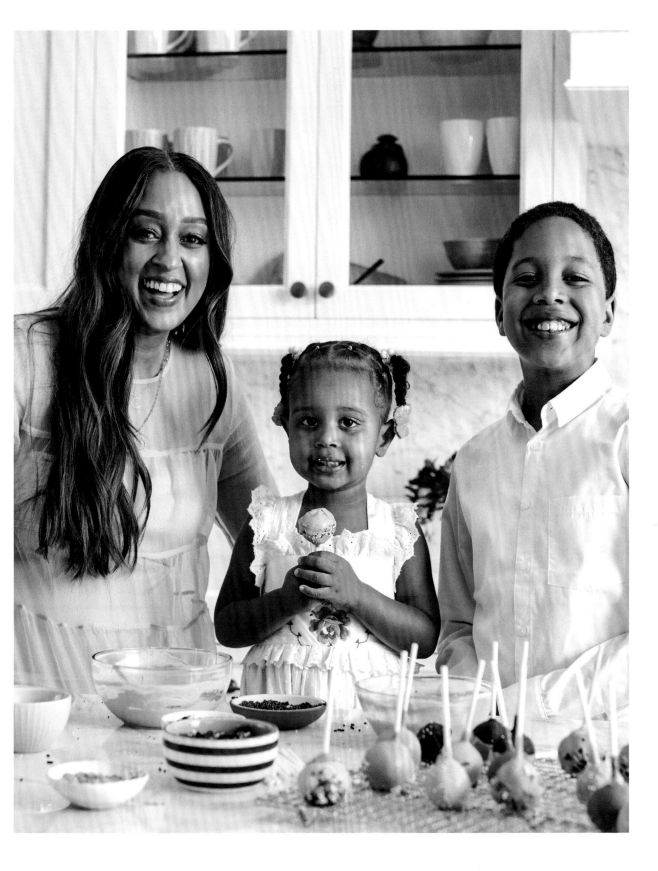

dinner—one I made from start to finish—meant I contributed something solely mine, which filled me with pride and ownership.

In college, I discovered the Food Network and devoured those shows incessantly. I studied Ina, Giada, Bobby, and Rachael and applied their wisdom in my own kitchen. When Rachael Ray used chicken broth to deepen a spaghetti sauce's flavor, it was a major revelation. How could something that straightforward have such a profound impact on a quick sauce? Her "30-Minute Meals" were packed with shortcuts and quick fixes, and that one tip inspired my journey to recognize when to veer from the pages of cookbooks and add my personal touch to dishes. From that day on, I always stocked broth or bouillon in my pantry . . . and had a knack for finding shortcuts, of course!

Ina Garten. Oh, I wished I was cool enough to be a guest at her table! I admired how she walked into her garden to snip fresh herbs, placing them delicately in her basket before crafting whatever grand feast lay ahead. I had a garden as well, but Ina made it all look so easy, and that motivated me to make the act of cooking—from tending to my own herbs, meal planning, and grocery shopping to preparing—a breeze. Watching her reminded me of family: her entertaining flair and setting the table for any occasion, serving everything family-style, and urging her guests to dig in! Do you notice every meal is an event for her? Even a modest get-together holds meaning! Mostly though, how sweet is her relationship with her husband, Jeffrey? She dedicated an entire cookbook to his favorite dishes and always makes sure he is well-fed with a smile on his face! Observing their interactions and her desire to nurture him with food was an example for Cory and me when we first became a couple. One day, I just knew Cory would be *my* Jeffrey. And look at him now! My Jeffrey!

Then there's the Italian beauty Giada who whirled pesto, dressings, and other charms in a food processor, folded the perfect ravioli, and maintained a flawless manicure through it all. She taught me how cooking honors your heritage and tells a story, whether from your own experiences, your ancestors', or your culture. And she stuck to her Italian roots with such conviction. When she pronounced every Italian word with gusto? I ADORED that. *Man-gia-mo!* (That means "Let's eat!")

My Food Network education drifted into my dreams. I used to wake up in the middle of the night with a flurry of ideas, which, of course, further intensified my obsession. I'd ask myself, "Tia! Girl, is this normal?" And depending on the day, I wondered if it was, in fact, normal. But my internal dialogue always saved me and responded with an enthusiastic "You know it!" Cooking was literally my dream. People make careers sharing and thinking about food, so why couldn't I? Well, as it turns out, dreams do come true! I got my own Food Network show, *Tia Mowry at Home,* and joined the ranks of my food idols! I even sat next to *the* Giada on a flight once, pinching myself the entire time to see if I was dreaming and holding back fangirl comments.

Anyway, when cooking for TV, they teach you how to provide context to the recipes. Specifically, sharing vignettes from the past that were attached to a memory or that inspired the dish. This type of storytelling helps engage the viewer, adds context, and provides an emotional attachment to the food. My show allowed me to cook (one of my favorite pastimes, duh) and share *me* on camera. Most of my fans knew me only as an actress on *Sister, Sister* and *The Game*, but on my cooking show, I expressed the real Tia. And that felt good. Finally, I was able to give you a glimpse into who I was as a real person. On TV, I invited friends and family to play with me in the kitchen. Teaching, rather than just cooking, became a completely different skill. I fully embraced the storytelling and recollections of my life directly associated with food, and I realized cooking for family and eating with them was a big part of my heritage. One of my favorite episodes featured my Caribbean background and cooking my aunt Blondie's heirloom curry chicken and potatoes. She and my cousin sat down with me as guests, and although I felt awfully nervous serving my interpretation of *her* dish, I also felt giddy to show her how much I valued what she had taught me. I cherish that episode because it was personal and gave me the chance to share that part of my history with a bigger audience.

When *Tia Mowry at Home* ended after three seasons, I desperately wanted to continue cooking on camera. If you've seen me cook, you know how much fun I have, even when

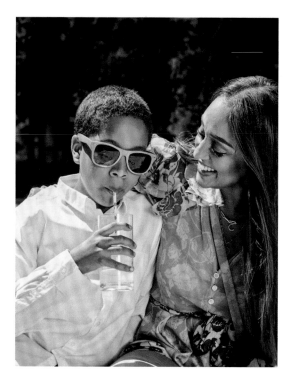

things are slightly off track. That's real. I am no different when the camera is off! I teamed up with Kin Community and we launched *Tia Mowry's Quick Fix* on YouTube, where I feature my everyday cooking, lifestyle and beauty tips, and lighthearted moments with my family. These videos are about more than putting food on the table. I'm sharing my trusted life hacks to support a more balanced, less overwhelmed day-to-day. On YouTube, I promote self-care and family time. If you feel good and are full of energy, then it's easier to radiate that to your loved ones. Aside from giving practical home-life advice and a peek into my world, I also want to empower you to eat at home with my fun and approachable recipes. Fitting cooking into your schedule establishes quality time and lets *you* choose the ingredients you and your family are consuming. Enter this book! I received a lot of enthusiasm from my viewers and wanted to give you all more access to my kitchen, recipes, tips, and tricks.

And like my last book, *Whole New You*, the *Quick Fix* mentality illuminates the importance of putting real food on the plate and doing good for *you*. By assembling meals for and with your family, you're providing valued sustenance and little souvenirs to carry through life. Food has longevity and encompasses the experiences, conversations, and emotions shared around the table. You know that saying, "The best way to the heart is through the stomach"? I obviously take that to the extreme, and I am not ashamed of it! Putting a home-cooked meal on the table is an expression of love. A meal, whether with my family or friends, is a celebration of togetherness.

I equate cooking to nurturing. Growing up, I did that for my siblings and parents. When I started cooking for Cory, my priorities changed and it became a different type of nurture, one that fostered our relationship. When he eats something I've made, his face lights up and I see pure appreciation beaming from him. After becoming a mother to Cree, that priority shifted even more. Where I'd usually be able to set aside an entire evening to lounge around and take my time with a meal while slowly sipping wine, I suddenly had a little person who needed every ounce of my attention. Although it was a jolt at first, I quickly embraced my duty to feed Cree and do everything in my power to guide him to become a healthy young man. I felt this incredible urge to nurture in a new way and fully grasped what food meant from a mother's perspective. We need food to survive and grow, and when my babies were born, I carried the responsibility to provide that to them. It was an immense blessing to then care for Cairo. When I stopped breastfeeding her, a wave of sadness overcame me since I could no longer nourish her with milk. But luckily, that didn't mean I had to stop feeding altogether! As I did with Cree, I realized there are other ways: weekend pancakes, eggs, and sausages cut into little circles, just like my mom did for my siblings and me.

To me, family is EVERYTHING. Family keeps me motivated. Family is my foundation for tackling the world. Family is my support system. I am still anchored to my childhood memories when I cook dinners because every time I do, I'm retelling a story. That right there is tradition: conveying history through an act. Mealtime is a genuine way of sharing traditions. The pleasure I feel when I make my mom's collard greens and place them on the table, saying, "These are my mom's greens," is tradition. I want my kids to make MY greens for their kids and say the same thing! I purposely provide these little twinkles of love for my children because I want "My grandma made those BOMB biscuits" to be carried on for generations.

I want you to recall one of your favorite food memories. Think about the colors of the room, the weather outside, the fragrances that filled the space that perked you up with excitement. Who was there? What sounds surrounded you? Were you wearing something special or your PJs? Okay, now close your eyes and savor that memory. Got it? Allow me to share one of mine:

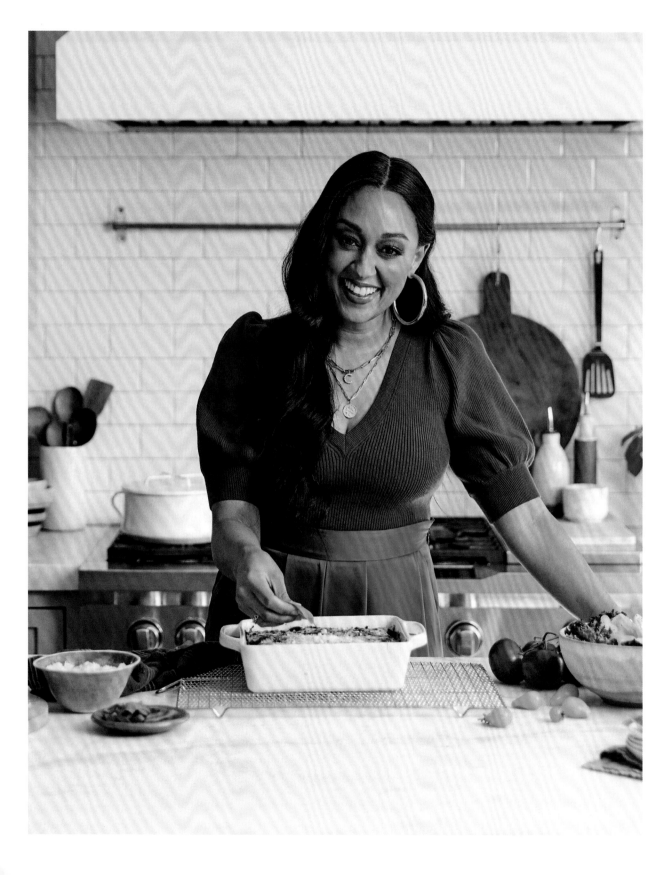

IN COLLEGE, I studied abroad with my sister in Florence, Italy. There, we witnessed food expressed in a new way. Beyond the flavors, textures, and fresh ingredients, I was introduced to a different way of life by way of food. Every weekend, Tamera and I traveled somewhere new and experienced all that the country had to offer. I tasted so many divine gelatos, pasta, meats, cheeses, and olives. A particular meal is forever embedded in my soul. On one getaway, we took the ferry to the island of Sardinia off the west coast of Italy. When we arrived, I vividly remember hailing a cab, and up pulled an old Mercedes-Benz driven by a female taxi driver. At the time, this was so curious because in Los Angeles or New York I only ever saw male drivers, and this woman looked like she was dressed up for an evening of dancing. She wore a flowy dress with a red scarf tied snugly around her neck, her hair perfectly messy. She had that effortless Italian confidence you see in movies. The car ride took us through windy and narrow roads nestled between olive and citrus groves.

Atop a hill sat a quaint restaurant the size of a shoebox, with a view extending to what felt like the length of the world. The ocean glistened with little diamonds dancing in the sun as we squished into our seats at a tiny table pushed up against the wall. After perusing the menu, which was in Italian, we asked the waiter to choose for us. He was delighted at the opportunity and ushered in a parade of food: first the little nibbles of cheese and shimmering olives, then a whole grilled fish with eyes, fins, and all. He methodically filleted it with a precision I'd never seen before, carefully extracting the bones before laying the flaky fillets on our plates. The delicate nature and glee he had while doing it captivated us, and everything after that continued to blow our minds. The simplicity was evident with each burst of flavor. Did they just catch that straight from the ocean? Pick the vegetables from a hidden garden? Pluck olives from a neighboring tree? There was no doubt in my mind that indeed they had done all of that.

After several hours of filling ourselves to the brim, we needed gelato. A slight breeze guided us to a *gelateria*. I chose my favorite two-scoop pairing—hazelnut and *stracciatella* (vanilla flecked with chocolate shavings)—and we plopped down side by side on a swing set. From there, we watched the villagers carry on with their day-to-day, while we contemplated if this was real life. It felt like heaven. After that, we hailed another taxi, this time driven by a cheery Italian man who proudly rattled off Sardinian facts in broken English. We were there only for a few hours, but the trip left an impression that will last a lifetime. Anytime I order a whole fish (typically branzino), I go right back to that tiny table with my sister.

What made it so beautiful and unforgettable was the freshness and purity of it all. Not just the air and the quaintness of our surroundings, but the food we savored. No bite felt overbearing. Instead, we tasted the food at its peak. Nothing overly salted. Nothing overshadowed anything. The balance of flavors allowed us to taste every component, every layer. In Italy, love is an ingredient, seen in the presentation and their enthusiasm. Their giving attitude (rather than take, take, take) enlightened me on how to provide food infused with passion and soul. Italians live to eat!

Taste and smell have the extraordinary ability to transport you through time. When I cook, I hearken back to my chapter there and try to bring that to my kitchen. Now back to you—how can you share your memory with your loved ones? It may not be with the same dishes or the people in the room, but is it possible to re-create the laughter and abundance that made it so special?

My intention with *Quick Fix* is to gift you my kitchen wisdom and hacks, so you have time to offer food as personal keepsakes, just like that memory. I want you to embrace the process so that it becomes second nature and flows effortlessly, like that waft of sweetness from the oven when freshly baked cookies are ready.

When you gather with your loved ones, you are sharing your passion and joy by enjoying the present moment together. This is what they'll remember and pass down.

I wrote this book with family in mind, providing hands-on ideas meant for getting the clan together. A tradition is difficult to make if everyone is in their room, so I encourage you to involve them in the process. That may not mean nightly. I don't know about you, but sometimes I need the kitchen to myself for a little namaste while I pound out some chicken and let go of that traffic jam I sat in for an hour longer than I should've. Kneading bread also helps with that, by the way!

But seriously—whether you're a new cook or someone who is looking to refine your skills and garner more insight from a busy bee like me, we could all use a little help. So, I've come up with recipes that are easy to make during a hectic workweek, using my favorite tips that have helped me sharpen my skills and allowed me to cook no matter what's on my calendar. For me, it's finding balance: in my schedule, in the flavors and textures of my food, in the dietary needs of everyone around the table, in the way I hold my knife. Once I'm balanced, I'm ready for takeoff. My goal is to smoothly juggle the components in order to bring it all together. If I drop a ball, well, I pick it up and fling it back into the mix. And hopefully, after reading this book, you'll be able to do the same.

A tradition is history being portrayed generation after generation; gifts to those who come after you; little blessings that help you relive moments time and time again. To express traditions you hold dear, or make new ones, is a tribute to life. I am passing down what my parents gave me, including having my son set the table and making sure that we authentically interact during mealtimes. My goal is to try to do this most of the time, despite our wacky schedules (and if I don't, that's okay! Thank goodness for leftovers!), holding utensils to enrich our bellies and our souls. I hope this book brings absolute joy into your home!

XOXO,
Tia

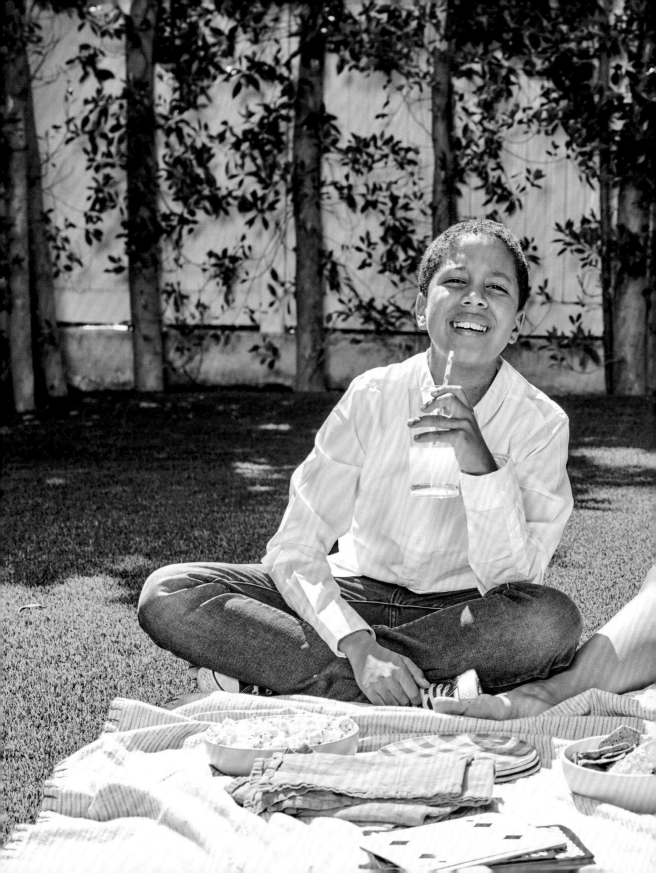

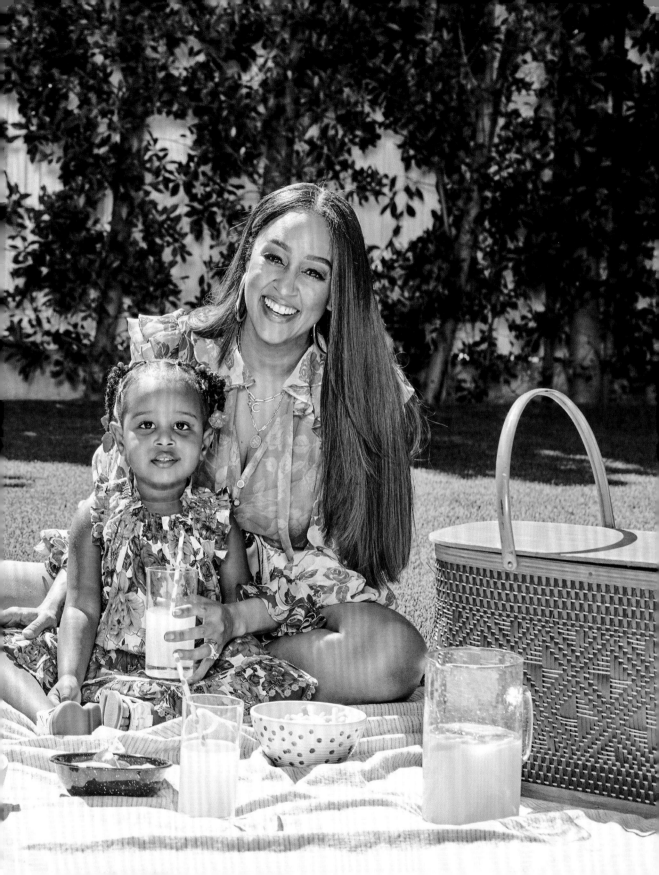

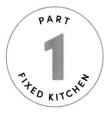

WHAT IS QUICK FIX?

quick ✦ adjective \ 'kwik \
acting or capable of acting
with speed: such as fast in
development or occurrence;
done or taking place
with rapidity; fast in
understanding, thinking,
or learning

fix ✦ verb \ 'fiks \
to repair or put
in order

The fact that you're reading this book means you want to cook, and I am PROUD. OF. YOU! If cooking isn't your thing, start small and get comfortable with your kitchen, knife skills, tools, and equipment. Familiarize yourself with the flavors that keep you going back to your favorite restaurant. Talk to the things in your kitchen like people talk to plants, why not? If anything, you'll get a hearty laugh out of it. A spatula will never talk back, so it's the perfect audience for a vent session!

Most people who shy away from cooking are scared that people will scoff at their food. I assure you right here and now, there's no need to impress anyone or be perfect. That fear is a stumbling block holding you back. Kick that block to the curb, and spread those carefree wings of yours. I am not going to teach you how to use tweezers to garnish a dish gently. No way. That is not my jam! I like making things look pretty, but you don't need to be an artist or executive chef with Michelin stars to serve a meal your family enjoys. Heck, you don't even need to be a chef! All you need is the willingness to seek out quality ingredients and put them together for whatever masterpiece works in your household. This may sound corny, but it is more important to serve love than a dish that took you three days to make. Cooking doesn't have to mean concocting elaborate meals like that. It can also mean blending a smoothie or tossing greens together for a salad. That, believe it or not, is cooking! Cooking is also an act of unwinding, loosening up, and singing as loud as you can while using your therapy spatula as a microphone!

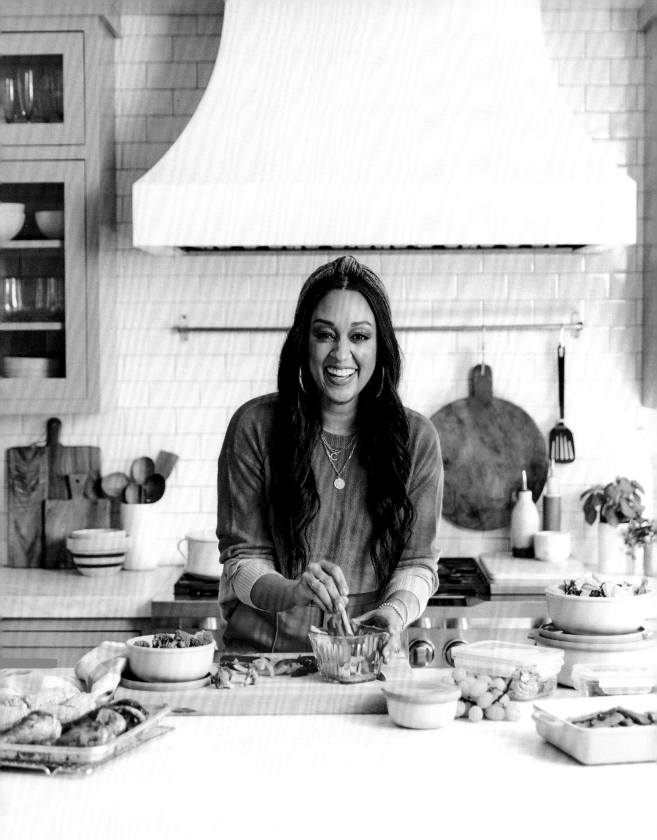

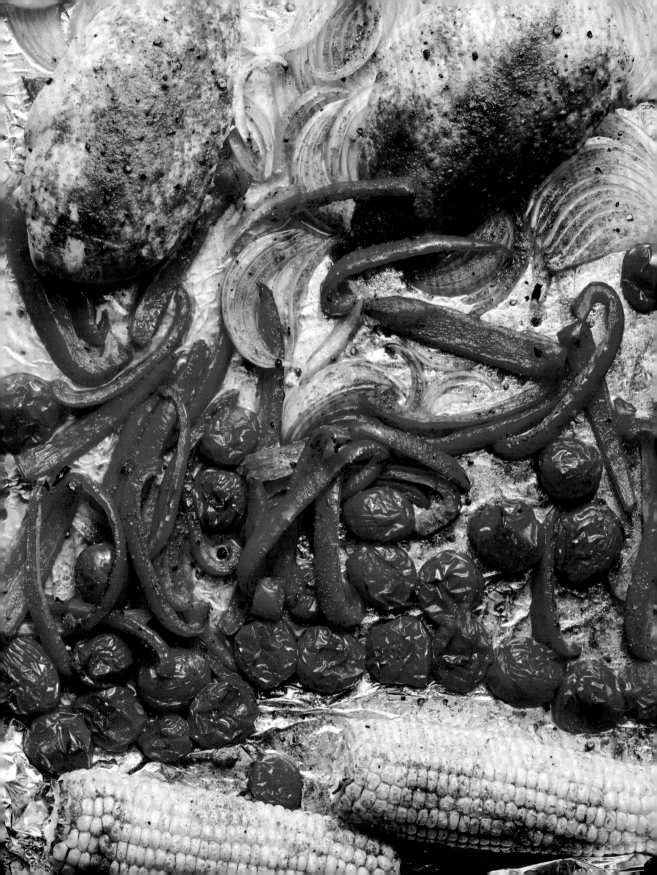

If you've seen *Tia Mowry's Quick Fix*, you know my style is a little bit of skill stirred with what's available, back to basics cooking, so it's easy (and enjoyable) to put dinner on the table even with a crazy life. I want to make that task accessible and enjoyable for everyone. I am a busy mommy and value my career, but the kitchen connects me daily to the people close to my heart. Since we need to eat, dinner is the natural means to integrate togetherness into our daily hustle. I couldn't do it with overcomplicated, laborious recipes! Therefore, I achieve that togetherness by sticking to the easy stuff and adding a bit of my personality.

As you can probably tell, I am very inspired by my mom. This book is, too. She rarely meal planned or jotted down extensive grocery lists. She made do with whatever was in the kitchen because she's an on-the-fly superwoman. She floated around with little means and never complained about it. Remember that show *Door Knock Dinners* where chef Gordon Elliott went into people's homes and assembled a marvelous banquet with whatever tidbits they had in their pantry and fridge? It's that type of improvisational cooking my mom did for our family: learning which herbs and spices go together, knowing standard roasting times, laughing at blunders, and appreciating whatever ended up on the plate. Our kitchen was that basket from *Chopped*: What can we make right now with canned green beans, frozen chicken breasts, and gummy bears? Voilà! A feast! As I've grown into my own cooking style, I've mingled my mom's ingenuity with my own. I lean on whole ingredients and try my best to eliminate additives, preservatives, and all the icky stuff in processed foods. Because of this, I *do* find meal planning a vital piece to the puzzle. Doing so keeps me organized with only one trip to the grocery store a week. By having my passion and process in place, I can fulfill weekly meals more efficiently.

Again, food is our means of survival. Back when our ancestors had to hunt and gather, the tribe sat together to partake in the bounty brought to them. Eating sustained their bodies. While we don't go to such extremes to eat nowadays, it has become difficult to assemble the tribe and give our bodies wholesome foods. To accomplish both, I focus on whole foods and recipes with easy-to-follow steps. Take lasagna: Instead of boiling the noodles, laying out the noodles, and trying to keep them from sticking together while I'm wrangling my daughter, Cairo, I use ravioli (cheese inside a noodle pillow) and put everything in a baking dish without all those steps, but with the same delicious result.

Quick Fix is playful. It aims to transform what might be a chore into something you adore. And if you already find pleasure in cooking, it's a way to amplify that love. Cooking is therapeutic to me. I'm either fully present when measuring ingredients or letting go of stress by concentrating on vigorously chopping herbs. Look, I'm no Mary Poppins. My purse isn't filled with a playground of necessities to make life effortless, but I do have some tricks up my sleeve and that inner Mary Poppins song and dance. *Quick Fix* finds balance for your family and the food you eat, and (you know me) sparks fun while doing it. Rather than watching the water come to a boil as the clock ticks down, I put the music on blast and cook like no one is watching! If your kid is by your side, play "Let It Go" for the thousandth time and yell that song for the neighbors to hear. Getting a noise complaint is just a minor setback. Find your groove! Some days it feels like there aren't enough hours to accomplish everything. But when I'm with my family in the kitchen and around the table, time seems to disappear.

Splash sauce on these pages. When you pass it down to your kids, they'll see memories in those spills, and whether or not they remember it as a mistake or remnants of a special meal, I'm sure they'll smile. Let's open up the cabinets, spruce them up a little, stock them with the necessities, and reveal the gems of your kitchen!

THE IMPORTANCE OF FOOD

My food choices supply me with the energy I need to get from morning to night, tackling all the duties in between. When eating, the body breaks down food molecules so they can be easily absorbed and converted into energy. Those vital nutrients and minerals then travel throughout this complex machine of ours to build muscle tissue, sustain organs, and power the body's survival mechanisms that are necessary to thrive. To be the best mom I can be, the wife I want to be, the friend I hope to be, the daughter, the sister, the colleague, and the writer of this book, I need to eat, and eat well, for my body and mind to function. My children also need to eat to grow and develop into people who give to the world. The great thing is, food is enjoyable! Food is GOOD! It's a delight to the palate, heart, and soul, and it's a significant component of human existence.

Modern-day life is fast-paced and requires a quick response. Time is often limited, but that doesn't erase the fact that food is yummy fuel. With short attention spans and rapid-moving schedules, a quick fix is a great way to supply us with life-affirming needs. So, when I say "quick," I mean quick. The clock is always ticking, and while people say we all have the same number of

hours in a day . . . do we really? Some days, it certainly doesn't feel that way. That's when I put on my speedy cape and do all I can to finish the job fast and easy! Since time is of the essence, these pages honor those precious minutes by helping you better understand the basic foundations of cooking—holding a knife properly and learning flavors—and cutting back on prep and cleanup to give you more time around the table. Each recipe is to the point because if I ever see an ingredient list longer than movie credits, I keep walkin'! And while I enjoy making exotic dishes every once in a while, scouring the city to find a rare root powder isn't something I can do all the time. Nor are those specialty ingredients accessible to everyone.

I use "fix" to help you get your kitchen in tip-top shape so you, too, can float through it like me and my mom. Yes, these recipes are designed for quick preparations, but the book itself is a fix that makes cooking approachable. If you and the kitchen aren't buddy-buddy quite yet or you don't have time to cook but desperately want to use it as a tool of engagement with your friends and family, this is a fix. And if you just need a boost because you're scraping the bottom of the barrel for new, healthful recipes suitable for your schedule, then here's the fix for that, too! If you feel like the quality of your meals has gone down as your responsibilities have gone up, this is a fix. Throughout this book, you'll discover quick fixes and little pearls of wisdom I use daily. This is my recipe box of home cooking with the little notes from my journey: advice from my mother, mentors, other cookbooks, friends, and the ever-present trial and error!

I have an open kitchen with an island so that even when people aren't hands-on helping, they're still a part of the experience. While I stir a stew and Cory talks to Cree about his day, I can turn around and insert myself into the conversation (whether they like it or not!), engaging every step of the way. It makes me feel like I'm entertaining, even if my special guests are just my family. If you don't have an island that allows a group effort, know that you can also prepare some of these recipes around a table. With the Baked French Toast (page 134)—a riff that combines torn bread with accoutrements in one baking dish—you can do the mixing and melding together.

This is all about finding balance in your life and the food you eat, from the little indulgent comforts, healthy necessities, and the tasty treats that always have the family running to the kitchen in a hurry. When cooking at home, you're in control of what you and your family consume for energy. I prefer my kitchen most of the time for several reasons:

BUILDING TRADITIONS. Research shows that dinner conversation elevates a child's storytelling, word comprehension, and relationships. I know I'm repeating myself here with the importance of traditions (and this isn't the last time, believe you me), but storytelling and creating narratives are what life is all about. Thousands of years ago, our ancestors found ways to relay their tales to us by scribing pictographs on cave walls. The act of dinner conversation has a similar effect.

WHAT'S IN THIS DISH. Knowing what my family and I are eating is top of the list, second to traditions. Today, a lot of restaurant chefs pride themselves on locally sourced ingredients, which is terrific! Knowing where our food comes from and understanding the environmental conditions in which it is cultivated is vital in making healthy choices for our bodies and our world. Cooking at home gives me this control every day. I can make the choice among processed foods, ethically raised meats, and portion control. You can better evaluate sodium levels, caloric intake, and preservatives that might be in your meal at home. It wasn't until recently that chain restaurants started putting nutritional data on their menus, which I think threw a wrench in some beloved favorites and had me second-guessing a lot of what I had been eating for years without even knowing the real nutritional implications.

EATING LESS. Even if you're mindful of portion sizes at restaurants, you may not realize you're eating more there than at home (oftentimes, three times more!). It's a special outing after all, and I know as long as that plate is sitting there, I'll likely pick at it until it's disappeared.

MONEY SAVER. Restaurants are integral in our culture. Anytime I go to a restaurant, I am in awe and inspired by the creations dancing through the joyful atmosphere. The flip side is the check at the end of that experience. If I do the math on my grocery bill, the cost per person averages $4 to $6 depending on the protein (because that's where there's an uptick). At a restaurant, we're lucky to leave with less than $12 per person, and that's a kid's meal! Not to mention the upcharge on wine or cocktails. So, imagine the money saved if you swapped the dine-out-to-dine-in ratio.

SPENDING MORE TIME TOGETHER. When I studied abroad in Florence, I noticed that the staff at restaurants never rushed us through a meal. Hours flew by in a blink. In America, most restaurants have "turns," meaning different time slots for reservations. Doing so helps streamline the kitchen for a steady flow in and out. Your meal has a time limit. At home, there is no time limit. No rush to finish up and move on. Add in the time spent cooking together, and you have an entire evening of bonding! This may not always be the case for kids with a lot of energy or homework, but on those days where you want to pamper yourself with a glass of wine, slouch down just a tad in your chair, and remain still until you're about to nod off? You have that at home. Bonus? Licking your plate clean! Just kidding, I don't do that. (Yes, I do.)

USING THIS BOOK

Writing this book has been a pure joy. I've transported to my childhood to revisit moments that shaped me into the cook I am today. I've recalled memories by simply plunging into the idea of homemade tacos like we did every Tuesday as a kid. I've inspired myself to keep going and cook regardless of how overwhelmed I feel, because cooking grounds me in a way I hope it does for you.

I wrote this book specifically to bring people around the table and devour the endless perks of eating as friends and family. In *Whole New You,* I detailed my journey through endometriosis and the healing powers of food. While *Quick Fix* isn't a health book, per se, uniting everyone to talk, love, and eat is healthy for the soul. By providing simple recipes that cover all genres—delectably indulgent and purely healthy—you will save time and allow space for family time, no matter the occasion.

Within these pages, we'll be honoring food and our health, creating memories, and going full throttle in the kitchen. If you're not jumping out of your seat excited yet, then huddle up with the team to designate and share the duties. Perhaps start with "You cook, I clean." Or "I cook, you clean." When everyone is involved—from meal planning, cooking,

setting the table, and wiping that last spill before digging into dessert—it takes some of the pressure off your shoulders.

This book is here to help you. It's your kitchen companion. And since I want to make things easier for you, I would suggest reading a recipe from start to finish before jumping in. Countless times, I've added all the ingredients at once, even though the recipe required it be done in different stages. Or, I accidentally added an ingredient twice because my head was somewhere else entirely. Sometimes you get lucky, and that accident works, but occasionally it doesn't (especially when it comes to baked goods!). One time while making cookies, the instructions said to microwave the butter for 10 seconds to soften. I somehow read it as "mix butter for 10 seconds," and not surprisingly, the cookies came out like bricks.

I also streamline the process by fetching the ingredients in one fell swoop and giving myself a pep talk. "Tia, this is it. It's dinner time. Ready, set, go, girl!" Then I turn on my music and enjoy the aroma that slowly begins to waltz throughout the house, signaling the family it's time to come down.

Like my last book, I've incorporated swaps that highlight the flexibility of these recipes. Most allow for substitutions to cater to any nutritional needs or make it accessible with whatever you have on hand or prefer. There is no need to stick to a recipe once you know the basics. I have a friend who never makes pesto because the conventional recipe calls for expensive pine nuts. After learning about this fraught relationship between pesto and him, I told him he could use any kind of nuts! Recipes aren't commandments set in stone. They are guidelines meant to inspire. With that said, look forward to the following types of recipes:

FUN. For those days you feel like a little indulgence, you'll find homemade pizzas, "brookies" (brownies + cookies = brookies), a creamy one-pot mac and cheese, all packed with tasty flavors, made simply. Monday through Thursday, I'm pretty strict about the food I eat, but I let go and treat myself to the fun ones on the weekend.

WHOLESOME. Recipes that focus on whole, fresh ingredients that also happen to be healthier, including a pasta Alfredo made with white beans (see page 212) that takes the classic dish for a spin, or the Super Nachos with Vegan Cheese Sauce (page 227) that is a constant in our household.

KID-FRIENDLY. Although most of this book can incorporate a kid-helper at some stage, several recipes are specifically designed for an all-in engagement at any age. Bring curiosity to the kitchen and use the space as a lab for tasty experiments.

Now, let's jump in to organizing your kitchen—an essential part of the *Quick Fix* process!

ORGANIZED KITCHEN

organized ≠ adjective
/ ˈȯr-gə-ˌnīzd / having
one's affairs in order
so as to deal with them
efficiently

I like to keep a well-stocked, tidy kitchen that helps rather than hinders. Strive for organization (from drawers, cabinets, and pantry) and make sure you own the appropriate tools to complete a dish. You don't need to overhaul everything and spend thousands of dollars on a kitchen remodel, but twice a year I evaluate my kitchen from top to bottom and see what's working or not. I find this brings peace to my space! Do you know why they tell you to make your bed in the morning? Because a messy bed sets the stage for a messy day. Every time you enter the bedroom and see untidy sheets, your subconscious tenses up. When the bed is made, you walk in and out of a place of serenity! I encourage that same technique in the kitchen. Arrange a tidy area where you'll *want* to cook.

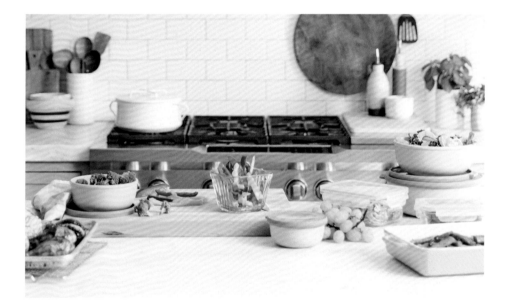

ORGANIZING

My cooking environment is cool (until I've got those burners on high!), calm, and collected. An organized kitchen can be your best friend, allowing you to gracefully move through the cooking process without searching every drawer for a tool or spice. Invest some time to declutter and organize now to avert a tizzy later.

DECLUTTERING

Remember a couple of years ago when the Netflix series *Tidying Up with Marie Kondo* took the country by storm, and everyone dug in and dug up their clutter? Donation centers across the nation saw a massive increase in contributions, and some even had to turn people away. Everyone clamored to tidy up after that show aired, and with good reason. While the process of cleaning and letting go can be emotionally and physically draining, it is ultimately immensely fulfilling. Often you don't realize that clutter is cramping your style or causing stress until you've slimmed and neatly arranged all your stuff. Once you do it, you'll see new potential for the space you're simplifying. This can provide flow in the kitchen, accessibility to the tools and ingredients you need, and a quicker run from start to finish. When I do this, I like to set aside a day where I can take the time to complete the task. Roll up your sleeves and filter through your current stock.

STEP 1: GET COMFY

I like to put on an outfit that allows movement (or I stay in my pajamas because nothing is cozier than that), sync my speakers, and play music that keeps me energized and focused. Or, if I haven't had my morning cup of brew yet, I pick a podcast or book that makes me concentrate. Sometimes, an entire hour will go by without my even noticing!

STEP 2: REMOVE

Whenever I declutter, I start by emptying the cabinets and drawers *completely*, laying everything out on the counters and table to see my inventory. If you need extra space, spread a blanket on the ground and place it all on the floor. Doing this gives you a clear view of what you own, so you can review everything at once when you diligently peruse it later on.

STEP 3: CLEAN

Give the empty shelves a good clean. It's not often there's a clean slate like this, and it's important to take advantage when there is one.

STEP 4: ASSESS YOUR GOODS

At this stage, I consider what I don't use or no longer need. Last time I did this, I found some crazy tools I *never* used, like slicers that serve *one* purpose and one purpose only: a banana slicer, tomato slicer, strawberry slicer, and an egg slicer. I'm not sure where or when I got them,

but I instantly knew where they were going (hello, donate pile!). These one-use gadgets take up more space than they're worth, and when you clear them away, wow, your kitchen can take a breath of fresh air!

During this step, focus on the essentials. You know the stuff you use often and things that make you happy when cooking. Anything that rarely (or never) sees the light of day? Do as Elsa does, and let it go. I compiled a list of my favorite tools (see page 41) to guide you through this. You will notice they are standard, back-to-basics stuff you may already have! Unless you are a ladle collector, there's no need for 27 different ladles.

STEP 5: SAY GOODBYE

I donate what is no longer of use to my family because it may be a treasure for someone else. You never know, a family up the road may cherish a banana slicer like a long-lost friend! If a tool or gadget no longer functions, feel free to throw it away.

STEP 6: ORGANIZE

Keep in mind, you are organizing to make your life as a home cook easier, so consider easy access, clean storage, and visibility.

After deciding what to keep and what to toss, place everything you are keeping back, but wait! Do it thoughtfully, with convenience in mind. I organize my kitchen to help me cook more efficiently. I consider how I cook and where I am when I need specific tools or spices. For instance, I typically need a spatula when I'm sautéing, so it has to go near the stove with the rest of my cooking utensils. Being intentional about arranging everything makes the cooking process smoother. Go online and you'll find affordable organizational fixes that work for you, whether that be matching airtight containers, supplemental shelves to optimize your cabinet and pantry space, separators for your drawers, or big mason jars for your bulk items. There are a ton of options for any kitchen that may inspire a total revamp or simple solutions! Here's how I do it:

Counter Space

If you have the room on the counter, go ahead and use it to your advantage. I place my most-used tools on the counter where they are readily available and part of my decor! My cutting boards lean against the wall; wooden spoons and spatulas stand proudly in a happy vase near the stove (you can also use a cute pitcher, which I think is adorable). My knives are snug in a drawer close to the action. Other everyday items, including my salt and pepper, are strategically placed for quick Salt Bae moments (if you're not familiar with Salt Bae, give it a quick search; the videos are ridiculous in the best of ways).

Cupboards/ Drawers

With items that don't end up on the counter, try categorizing them close to where they are used. For example, I keep my cooking utensils in the drawer nearest the stove and place oven mitts, trivets, and bakeware by the oven. My heavier appliances reside below the counter for safety purposes, along with pots, pans, mixing bowls, and other miscellaneous devices, such as my dearest food processor. Cups, plates, and other dishware go above. And kiddo plasticware can go in a drawer designated for them, so they feel like a big girl or boy when they pick out their plate.

If you don't have a dedicated food pantry, mingle canned provisions, starches, and other non-perishables together to better remember everything's place.

Storage

Mindfully storing brings happiness to your space. I prefer loading dried goods and bulk items (oats, rice, flour, cereals) in my own containers rather than clogging up my shelves with a jumble of packaging, which makes it untidy. This also keeps them fresher longer and stops little bugs from taking a dip in the ol' flour bag. Again, there are many affordable options online, and I think you might find the search invigorating.

CLEAR CONTAINERS. When I get home from the grocery store, I pour oats and other starches into clear containers and jars because, for one, it looks pretty, and two, I can instantly determine what I have in stock. It helps to glimpse into the pantry, see the jar of elbow macaroni, and know immediately if I need more. For items like millet or bulgur grains that I forget cooking directions for, I snip the label off the package and tape it to the back where it's handy. Of course, nowadays, I can google the instructions, but what fun is that? As I said, this organization tip looks sleek. And as a bonus, clear containers eliminate the question, "Where did I put that darn thing?"

Sometimes, we accidentally overstock and spend more money by purchasing something we already have, simply because we didn't see we already had it. If you have a general idea of your inventory through concise organization, finding what you need should be a fluid grab-and-go process. I make things visible to eliminate a time-consuming hunt every time I need something. I also tend to purchase the same items repeatedly, which makes knowing what to get intuitive.

AIRTIGHT. We all know that one drawer or cupboard packed with mismatched container lids and bottoms. It's refreshing when I set aside time and give that space attention. Go on, try it for yourself. Or have a kid do it for you! They love matching things together, and I'm sure they'll appreciate this "game." Use a lonely bottom as an organizing tool (if it's big enough, you can put fruit snacks or other small items in it) or recycle it. Say a loving goodbye to the things that no longer serve a purpose.

FIXED PANTRY

Having everything ready to go when you need it is the truest quick fix of them all: basic ingredients on hand, key tools to actualize the meal, and a cheery attitude (more on this in a moment). Even if your pantry looks a little bare now, once you start working your way through this book, you'll have everything you need at your fingertips because there is a lot of overlap in the ingredients used.

This gives you the ability to cook on the spot whenever required of you or your partner, or your kids if they're old enough to take charge. I'm giving you a list that works for my family and makes nightly dinners accessible for us, no matter the schedule preceding it. Review and adjust according to your household. Here's a quick starter:

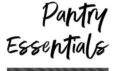
Pantry Essentials

TIA'S TRINITY: Onion, garlic, extra-virgin olive oil
If you have Tia's Trinity on hand, you're straight. You're good. You can make something delicious, even if the rest of your kitchen is lookin' slim. How many times have you read "In a skillet, heat oil over medium heat. Add onion and garlic and sauté until softened"? These three staple ingredients are the beginning of the best dishes across the globe. Your kitchen may feel left out of the party if it doesn't have them.

Olive oil tip: When purchasing olive oil, reach for extra-virgin types in dark-colored bottles. Olive oil will spoil or sour if exposed to light or heat over an extended period. And on that note, keep it in a dark, room-temperature place (not over the stove or oven).

KID'S TRINITY: Pasta, butter, cheese
Let's face it, almost everybody, especially the little nuggets, loves plain pasta coated with butter and sprinkled with a delicate dusting of cheese. On those nights when your energy is at zero, it's time to have a plain pasta celebration! Go with whatever pasta

suits your needs—gluten-free, zucchini noodle, regular noodles—and fill up the bowls!

Pasta tip: Gluten-free pasta works almost flawlessly as a swap without too much adjustment. Follow the directions on the back of the box. Baked pasta may take some extra care but gluten-free noodles or lasagna sheets typically work as a replacement.

Butter tip: Grab unsalted butter for cooking and baking. This allows you to control your salt intake and steer clear of an oversalted meal.

OATS: Oats are an everyday go-to in baking and perfect for a fiber-filled breakfast for everyone in the family, quickly prepared the night before, so they're ready when you wake up. Oats are a great base to pile on fruits for an excellent start to the day! If your family is tempted by sugary cereals, have them try a cozy bowl of oatmeal sweetened with berries and bananas instead.

Oats tip: Opt for rolled oats over "quick" or "instant." Yes, I know we're going for quick here, and nothing is faster than an instant, but that variety has been processed so much it's virtually zapped of all nutrients. The good thing about rolled is you can prep it at night, so it's ready for the morning! Here's the oat tier, from least processed to most. When less processed, it does take longer to cook, mind you, but maintains most of its natural nutrients and fiber:

* Oat groats
* Steel-cut
* Rolled
* Quick

BREADS OR TORTILLAS: I tend to keep these lovelies in the kitchen at all times. Choose whatever variety suits your family's needs, because today's grocery stores carry many options, including gluten-free and grain-free varieties. Whatever you choose, I know that grilled cheese and quesadillas have come to the rescue more times than I can count! Great for quick snacks, lunches, or dinners.

MILK: If you scan the aisles of practically any grocery store, you'll see your typical cow's milk next to the alternative-milk squad. If they're not in the refrigerated section, the alternative choices are often in the cereal or baked goods aisle. I have a variety in my fridge—regular milk for Cree, Cory, and Cairo, and almond for me.

Alternative milk tip: It's pretty impressive how many milks are on the market now: nut (almond, hazelnut, cashew), soy, coconut, hemp, rice, and oat, to name the familiar bunch. I opt for "unsweetened" but if I'm looking for a sweet peck on the lips, I add agave to temper my sugar intake.

CHEESE: For those grilled cheese sammies and quesadillas, you gotta have the cheese! I get preshredded, whole-milk cheeses for quick lunches or after-school snacks.

PROTEINS: I don't usually buy more than I need for a particular week's meals, but I *do* purchase quality products: organic, farm-raised, grass-fed, no added hormones, and no antibiotics. I cover this more in the coming section, but know that quality proteins reduce the burden of chemicals (added hormones and antibiotics) from highly processed meats that sneak their way into your body. If you're opting for a seafood meal, look for wild-caught or certified farm-raised fish. More on this later, too.

SNACKS: I make sure we have little nibbles on hand to get through the day. The supermarket has a lot of health-conscious snacks available for the choosing! For packaged kids' snacks, I stock up on no-sugar turkey jerky, crackers, puffs made with lentils or chickpeas, crunchy can't-just-have-one dehydrated snap pea crisps, non-GMO popcorn, deli turkey slices, and fruit snacks made with real fruit juice. In the summer, my fridge is filled with berries and stone fruits (peaches, nectarines, plums, apricots), and during fall and winter, we load up on apples, bananas, pears, and carrot sticks.

PRODUCE: I look for what's in season, snackable, and fresh. In today's world, most produce is available year-round, but shopping during peak seasons assures freshness and optimum flavor. If you see something way out of season—peaches in winter—that means they probably traveled across the globe to get to you, or they're genetically modified organisms (GMO). If genetically modified, the plant's molecular structure has been manipulated to speed up harvest, or allow it to grow in varying climate conditions, where it usually would not. GMOs are a result of supplying the demand of our increased population. While GMOs help feed a great many people, the health impact is still unknown.

DRIED HERBS AND SPICES: I can't stress enough how much I use dried herbs and spices; they save me time on prepping and are always there for me. Using them also sidesteps the kids' Q&A about what "the green stuff" is on their plate when I add parsley or cilantro to a dish. I do a deep dive into the spice rack on page 78 to help ramp up your flavor knowledge!

Tip: Spices are at their best when stored in a cool dark place with an airtight lid. After buying a new spice, write the date on it, and you will never question how long you've had it. Spices (cayenne, paprika, curry powder) last two to three years, while dried herbs (oregano, thyme, bay leaf) hold on for one to two. To check if spices are old, place a little in the palm of your hand, rub it with your finger, then give it a whiff. If it's still good, the fragrance permeates and reminds you of something delicious. If the aroma or color is dull, it's time to go.

MISCELLANEOUS: These are the random most-used provisions constantly on rotation in my pantry. Always look for low- or reduced-sodium versions so *you* can control your salt intake:

✳ Vegetable or chicken broth: To add depth of flavor in a short amount of time. I will often use broth instead of water in my rice. If I'm sautéing cauliflower or broccoli, I may add a splash to help it along and give a little zing. Or if I'm cutting back on calories, I'll replace olive oil with room-temp broth in a pesto.

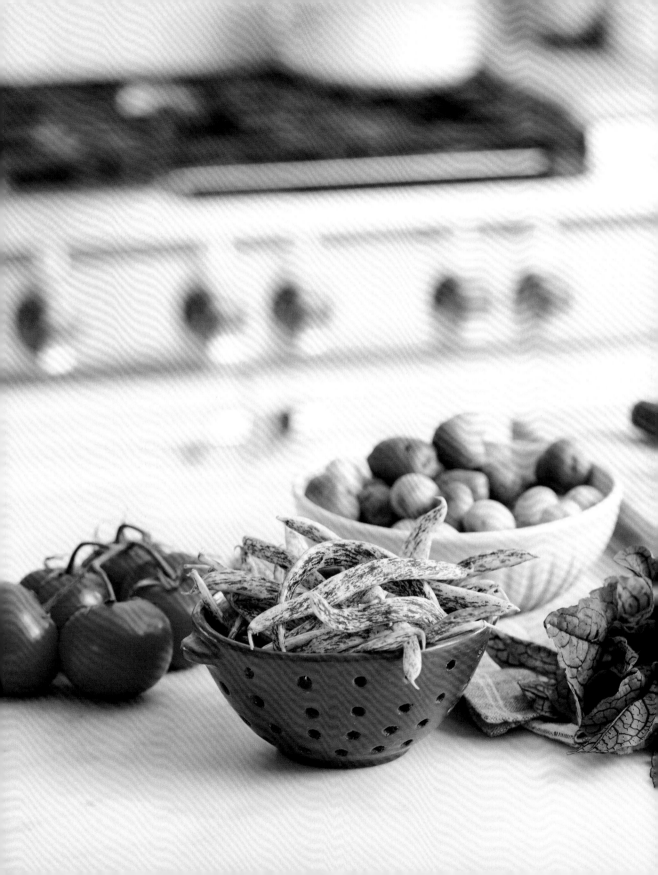

* Soy sauce or tamari: Both are made of fermented soybeans, but tamari eliminates the wheat used to produce soy sauce. If you're gluten-free, look for tamari and read the label to double-check that it is 100% wheat-free. Making a stir-fry is relatively easy (see Shrimp Stir-Fry with Cabbage, Scallions & Snap Peas, page 211) because it's a one-pan wonder, and after you familiarize yourself with the basic steps, you can make it anytime with any veggies you have in your fridge as long as you have soy sauce or tamari.

* Canned beans: Chickpeas, white beans, black beans: You'll find use out of these any time of the year, whether you're making a quick chili, an Alfredo with beans instead of cream (see Creamy "Alfredo" Pasta, page 212), or a cold summer salad tossed in a light vinaigrette. Beans are always handy and pack a robust helping of protein and fiber. Beans are typically the only canned items I carry in my pantry.

* Grains: Brown rice, quinoa, freekeh, millet, bulgur, barley: Guilt-free starches help balance any meal.

* Oils: Sesame, olive, avocado, grapeseed: Each serves a unique purpose because they vary in flavor intensity and smoke points (the temperature at which the oil starts to burn). Some oils (vegetable, canola, and safflower) have a high smoke point, which make them good for frying. Olive oil, on the other hand, starts to burn at a low temperature, so it's best for sautéing.

* Baking soda and baking powder: Essentials for baking, and you will notice they are used quite frequently throughout this book.

* Vanilla extract: Another principal baking need. Look for "pure" on the label!

PARCHMENT PAPER AND ALUMINUM FOIL: I use parchment and aluminum foil on top of my baking sheets for nonstick needs and easy cleanup.

TOOLS

Since I spend so much time in my kitchen, I've learned what equipment works best for me. I especially appreciate double-duty tools, like my box grater, which I employ to grate cheese, flake cold butter for a pie crust, and finely shred carrots or onions. Seldom am I managing 15 tools at once. The only time that many items are out is when Cairo decides to give a concert with the pans. I'm a one-sheet-pan type of gal. Spread the ingredients in a layer, stick it in the oven, watch the end of *Moana* even though I've seen it 1,500 times, and scroll Instagram while it's doing its thing.

Must-Haves

Kitchen innovation has absolutely found its way into the future, creating quite the population of gadgeteers in the process. Yet, some things just aren't necessary (ahem, hot dog slicer). Most kitchens already have the items on my list, but you may see some curious bits and bobs below that you haven't considered a necessity.

Knives

Sharp knives are paramount when cooking. I cannot stress this enough! When your knife is well-tuned and maintained, you will cut, chop, and slice a lot snappier. A dull blade won't get you anything except potential moments of frustration and a possible injury. If you are struggling with a dull knife, it can easily slip and nick your finger.

CHEF'S KNIFE: An 8- to 10-inch chef's knife will do most of the work around your kitchen, and if sharp, can do the work of all the knives.

PARING KNIFE: These blades typically run between 3 and 4 inches and are best for soft ingredients, like fruits and mushrooms, but are also great for the little guys like shallots and garlic. These are the knives you see grandmas use as they sit at the table, peeling apples and garlic in their hands with the grace of a classical guitarist.

SERRATED KNIFE: You may think this friend is used only for loaves of bread, but I use it to help me "saw" through the tough-rind ingredients, such as watermelon, winter squash, pineapples—and sometimes even tomatoes if I haven't had a chance to sharpen my chef's knife in a while. It's also suitable for peeling rinds off lemons and limes and trimming pie crust, or finessing the edges of a cake when I'm decorating like a boss.

Silicone Spatulas & Tongs

Aside from the general flat metal spatula well known for flipping pancakes, I suggest stocking your drawers with heat-resistant silicone-tipped spatulas. These helpers gently glide through a soft scrambled egg (see page 135) and pick up every ounce of food from your mixing bowls and skillets. Furthermore, they do not scratch your equipment's surfaces the way a wooden or metal spatula would. But just because they clean every inch of cake batter left over in the bowl doesn't mean you can't sneak a taste with your finger.

Silicone-tipped tongs won't scratch the surface of your pots, pans, and sheet pans. This is a core tool for everyday cooking while also for caring for your other equipment. It also doesn't tear aluminum foil the way a metal one would when picking up items.

— **FLAT SPATULA**
— **ASSORTED SIZES OF SILICONE SPATULAS**
— **ASSORTED SIZES OF TONGS WITH AND WITHOUT SILICONE TIPS**

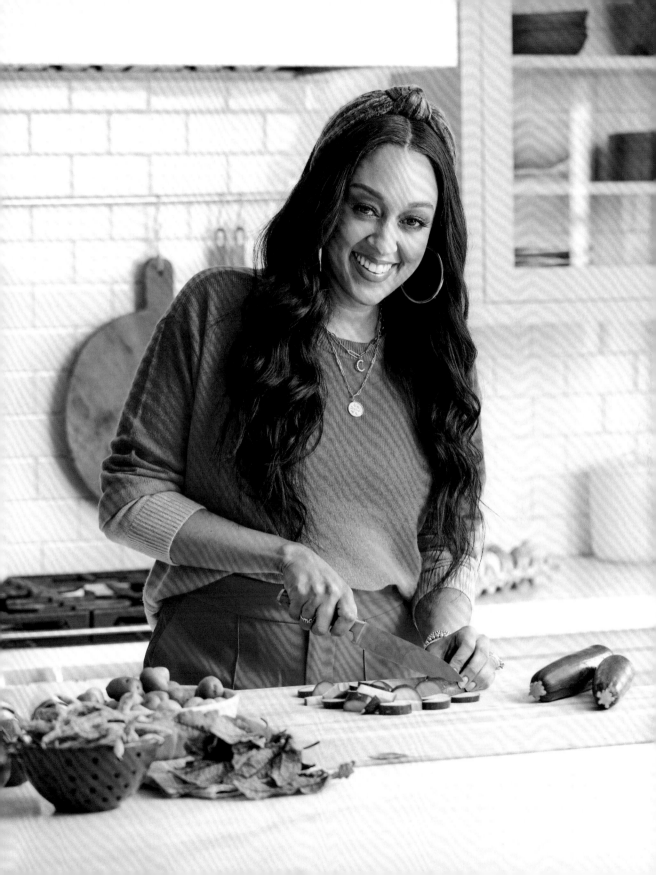

Spoons

These four major spoon styles will get you through any recipe, and I recommend a variety because of the unique purposes they serve. Aside from a wooden spoon, I choose metal because they last longer than the hard plastic ones, and if the plastic isn't BPA-free, those toxic chemicals may leach into hot soups, stews, or other steeping dishes. Metal allows you to wash in the dishwasher without warping. Just be careful not to aggressively scrape the bottom of your pans.

WOODEN SPOONS: These neither retain heat like a metal spoon, nor chemically react to acidic foods like tomato sauces. They also allow you to scrape the yummy bits on the bottom of a pan after braising.

METAL LADLE: Great for soups, stews, layering sauces in a dish like a lasagna, and pouring heaps of leftovers into plastic baggies or airtight containers without causing a spill.

METAL SPOONS: Good for general stirring. Not much to see here, but a kitchen requirement nonetheless.

METAL SLOTTED SPOON: The slots help drain off excess liquid when serving or can be used as a nifty sieve if you're transferring large noodles or ravioli from boiling water directly into a sauce.

Pots & Pans

An assortment of the main pots and pans will help you usher in every type of dish you want to cook, and the following are the perfect vessels for whatever you're whipping up, whether it's soups/stews/chilis, sauces, veggies, or omelets, and everything in between. Also, no toddlers' band is complete without this drum set, right?

10-INCH SKILLET (NONSTICK OR STAINLESS STEEL): The perfect tool for fluffy eggs or omelets, skin-on proteins, or general use. This size will get you through basic needs.

SAUTÉ PAN WITH LID: Great for stir-fries and other dishes that involve a hefty amount of ingredients. Using the lid will help trap moisture to steam a dish to perfection rather than adding more oil.

STOCKPOT, 8-QUART OR LARGER: I bring this puppy out for big-batch one-pot wonders, like stew, macaroni and cheese, stocks, and a variety of full meals made solely with this and only this. I have an entire section of recipes dedicated to this VIP (Very Important Pot).

SAUCEPAN, 3- OR 4-QUART: Valuable when warming smaller portions, melting butter or coconut oil, and swirling together a sauce.

Bakeware

You will see in the recipes that I cannot live without these two tools. They can accommodate big family meals, with minimal cleanup. My favorite type of meal is one where you can combine everything and then toss it into the oven. Without these, I'd be lost!

— **9 × 13-INCH BAKING DISH**
— **SHEET PANS**

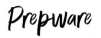

Prepware

I'm guessing you may already have these everyday pals. If not, then add them to your wish list!

WHISK: In addition to the obvious, it's also good for whipping warm milk into a nice frothy cloud for a homemade cappuccino.

VEGETABLE PEELER: Not just for the peels! Shave vegetable ribbons to top a salad or make wide zucchini noodles. Also use for shaving chocolate onto the top of brownies, pudding, a celebratory cake, and so much more.

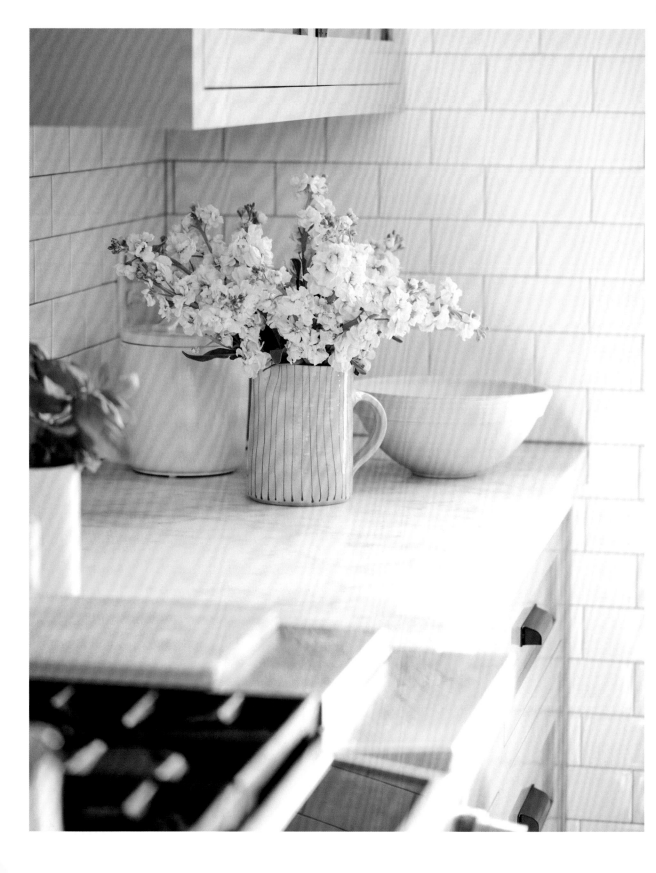

MEASURING CUPS/SPOONS: Both the cups and the spoons come in sets with different quantities. Aside from measuring, you can use the bottoms of the cups to trace circles for baking needs or to press down firmly onto something that requires flattening.

LIQUID MEASURING CUP: The measuring cups above are used for dry ingredients (like flour), but to measure liquids, you need this type of (usually glass) cup. Get one that holds 2 cups.

FINE-MESH SIEVE: Great for sifting, draining, straining soup stocks, or separating seeds from berries for dessert sauces or jams.

BOX GRATER: My go-to for grating and shredding onions, carrots, and other veggies into pieces that need to be small and equal in size. It's also an excellent hack to soften butter quickly. Rather than microwaving it, grate it into flakes, and it will come to temperature a lot faster.

MIXING BOWLS: Small, medium, and large: Size matters for baking because you'll typically need to mix dry ingredients separately from wet before their big marriage into the larger mixing bowl. I also use these for tossing and serving a big crunchy salad!

CUTTING BOARDS: Plastic or gel, and wooden: I prefer gel or plastic for cutting raw meats to avoid cross contamination. I bring out multiple cutting boards for proteins and other ingredients, and have colors for different things (i.e., red for meats, green for produce) to help me remember to keep raw meats separate. Because wooden cutting boards will soak up juices and harbor bacteria, save those for produce, cooked meats, cheese platters, or charcuterie.

KITCHEN TOWELS: I always have a kitchen towel over my shoulder, tucked in my apron, or in reach, because cooking can be messy, and a good wipe of the hands is always refreshing. I like cloth towels because they reduce waste.

Special Treats

These are the don't-need-but-must-haves specialty items. Once you and your kitchen have blossomed into a promising, happily ever after relationship, and you two darlings want to tackle more together, these are the little gifts that keep making life in the kitchen balanced.

8-INCH NONSTICK SKILLET: Because when it comes to kids, you're making quesadillas all the time.

10-INCH CAST-IRON SKILLET: Good for dishes that require a transfer from stovetop to oven. I sometimes make pizza in here!

9 × 9-INCH BAKING DISH: Used for cakes, corn bread, brownies, and dinner rolls.

DUTCH OVEN OR 6- TO 7-QUART HEAVY-BOTTOMED PAN WITH A LID: Distributes heat evenly. If you're not sure whether or not you already have this, look at your pot bottom. How thick is it? Is it heavy? These can get costly, so if you don't have one, use your stockpot and stir the dish from time to time, rotating the pan occasionally to even out the heat.

FOOD PROCESSOR (10- TO 12-CUP): A huge time-saver because it will do the chopping, mixing, and blending for you. Some also come with an attachment for grating vegetables, so if you're making carrot or zucchini muffins, this will be a time-saver. I use it for various recipes in this book, like Creamy "Alfredo" Pasta (page 212) and Quick Ranch Dip & Homemade Potato Chips (page 167). Throw 'em in, give it a whirl, and *ding!* It's done.

HAND MIXER OR STAND MIXER: When baking, both of these are crucial as they will do the beating and blending for you. Hand-whipped cream is ideal for upper arm strength, but it takes forever. Not when using an electric mixer!

BLENDER: The possibilities with a blender are as infinite as the night sky. Aside from blending a daily or nightly smoothie, it can whip a pesto into shape, a frozen banana into "ice cream," or fruits into Popsicle mix, as well as puree baby food if you make it yourself.

IMMERSION BLENDER: When blending soups, sauces, or other hot-dish items, this is an excellent gadget because you can blend things right in the pot rather than transferring them to a blender. I think of this as a special treat because it certainly is not a kitchen essential, but a quick fixer.

MEAT THERMOMETER: I highly recommend this because it is the trustiest indicator of when your poultry and other proteins are done—no one wants an under- or overcooked chicken. If you always desire juicy meats, invest in a meat thermometer. It will tell you whenever they're done without guessing.

ROLLING PIN: Just your standard pin. Nothing fancy here!

MICROPLANE: I debated whether or not to put this in the must-haves list! I use mine all the time to zest citrus (fresh lemon zest over steamed or roasted broccoli is YUM!), grate cheese, finely mince garlic or ginger (if I'm feeling under the weather, I simmer fresh ginger, water, and lemon juice to button me right up), shower chocolate shavings over Baked French Toast (page 134), or grate nutmeg for baking.

KITCHEN SHEARS: I use shears to open packaging, trim fat from proteins, cut pizzas and quesadillas, and snip fresh herbs and raw bacon (sometimes it gets a little fussy with a knife).

ICE CREAM SCOOPS (ASSORTED SIZES): Not just for ice cream! I use these to evenly scoop cookie dough and cupcake or muffin batter. Not as messy as a ladle or a spoon.

BENCH SCRAPER: No ingredient is left behind with a bench scraper. Using the sharp edge of your knife can lead to dulling of the blade and may scrape the plastic surface of a cutting board, which can get into your food.

BALANCED KITCHEN

balanced ∗ adjective
\ 'ba-lən(t)st \
taking everything into
account; fairly judged
or presented

This isn't a race; it's all about finding balance. When feeding yourself or a family, you balance numerous factors: proper nutrition the body needs to survive, requests that stem from a picky palate or an allergy, flavors, and techniques. Most important, you're balancing quality time for yourself with the people you love. It may seem difficult at first because knowing how to find the right equilibrium isn't necessarily innate. However, once you adapt to a system, you'll be like Simone Biles on the beam: getting on, gracefully moving through the routine, and dismounting with arms up, chest out, and a smile.

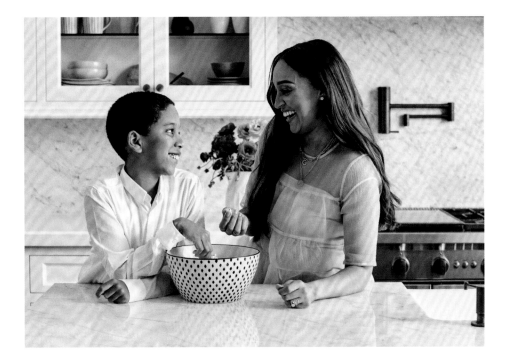

WHAT DOES "WELL-BALANCED" MEAN?

In *Whole New You,* my journey to decrease inflammation and recalibrate my digestive, immune, and reproductive systems led me to pregnancy and my girl Cairo. Learning about my diet—specifically how my body couldn't function under the weight of my unhealthy choices—changed my perception of food and ultimately my life. When I use the word "diet," I'm not referring to a trend everyone is following to lose weight. When I say "diet," I'm referring to the way I eat: the quality and composition of the food I consume daily. While shaped by my *Whole New You* journey, my current regimen is now a well-balanced mix of whole, healthy foods and a couple of indulgences that give me the warm fuzzies when I sit down to eat (even though they aren't necessarily "healthy").

I find indulgences necessary in life, as I do joyful experiences. So, for the sake of this book, know that "diet" is the lifestyle and choices made around food. Breakfasts, snacks, lunches, and dinners make up my diet, and while I'm not here to suggest a restricted set of guidelines, I personally balance each. The point is to support the helpers inside your body, keeping in mind that your body is continually working for you. In my life, it's in my best interest to champion that balance and work for *my body,* too. This philosophy helped me lose weight after the birth of Cairo at a pace that kept me sane and healthy. I didn't put pressure on myself to slim down quickly, I gave myself time and properly nourished my body while doing so.

How do I achieve a "well-balanced" diet for myself and my family? The term well-balanced means I am receiving my body's nutritional needs to bolster muscle tissue, energy, and cells that work every day to protect me. Our bodies are not tip-top without proper nutrition. When my diet is derailed, I become fatigued and can't perform the way I normally would if I'm eating well. Well-balanced nutrition affects a child's development, too, so I'm constantly exploring the best packaged snacks my kids eat. I won't get into the nitty-gritty here because each of us has a particular set of needs, each one of us absorbs or reacts to food uniquely, and each one of us requires a personalized diet for our individual bodies. But for all humans, a well-balanced lifestyle is influenced by access to food, preferences, family and cultural customs, age, time, and budget.

It seems like a lot to consider, but really, it's taking intuition to the next step: intention.

Know that everything counts: All food *and* drinks go through the digestive process. Quality and diversity in your diet matter. We need a wide range of essential nutrients to thrive so that good/helpful bacteria can act as Pac-Man to overpower and gobble up harmful bacteria that can lead to disease. These microscopic warriors, known as the microbiome, eliminate debris, keep the system in check, and help ward off potential illness.

Both the gut and its bacterial flora are crucial to overall health, from head to toe. For instance, the term "gut instinct" has an actual meaning: Our brain and gut are strongly connected, inseparable buddies that work closely together. We feel emotional responses in the gut because of the similar chemicals produced in both organs. If you experience extreme stress, you may get an upset stomach. Conversely, if the gastrointestinal tract is under repeated distress, the brain may falter. This is why gut health, and ultimately a well-balanced diet, is so important.

In recent years, you may have noticed chatter about the importance of a "diverse" microbiome, meaning a medley of good bacteria that aids in gut-health management. Think of it like a garden. A savvy green thumb will care for his or her flowers with proper nourishment and water. If the garden is neglected, it will fall into despair. Our microbiome is our garden, and our ancestors had a mightier one built by clean foods and nutrients. As we and our food system have evolved to implement processed chemicals and packaging, our microbiomes have become a bit weedy. According to an article in *Nature* magazine, lifestyle and environment can greatly impact the wellness of our individual microbiomes, including the foods and beverages we do or don't consume, excessive use of antibiotics (both in medication form and those absorbed through processed foods, like meats), and lack of fiber.

With this knowledge, it's clear that food is a vital piece to the puzzle. If I ate only junk food, my gut's systems would spend a lot of time breaking down and sorting out the unnatural additives rather than focusing on other necessary tasks. All of this could lead to inflammation and potential health complications. My precious microbiome would be overrun by the toxins from my wayward food choices. When this happens, I'm forcing my body to consider molecules not found in nature (preservatives and other additives) instead of the distribution of minerals needed. But by cycling in a rainbow of whole veggies, fibers, and proteins, I benefit from the wheel of vitamins (A, B, C, E, K, and so on) and minerals that promote cell growth and health, along with the diversity of my microbiome.

Let me tell you something: I've been caught in the twister of confusing, contradictory diet advice many times in my life, which is why I don't follow fleeting trends. I once cut out all fats from my diet because everyone said fats were bad, when in fact, good fats are good. Carbs? Those are not the enemy either! Fruits contain carbs, as do whole grains that supply essential nutrients. Balancing the food groups helps the various systems in the body function so we can walk, talk, laugh, and love.

To achieve a well-balanced diet, we need calories, a diverse selection of vitamins and minerals, antioxidants, carbohydrates (starches from whole grains and fiber), protein, and healthy fats. Together, these nutrients give you fuel so that all your systems are a GO. I do my best to avoid tipping the scale toward the naughty foods. I refer to the beautiful foods that should be front and center as "nourishing," since those are the foods that provide all that goodness to maintain balance in your body. The "indulgences" are those foods that I like to wiggle in when celebrating a long week, a birthday, or yearning for a decadent night!

Okay, so let's break this down: Nourishing foods provide the body with building blocks and these essential nutrients:

VITAMINS AND MINERALS: Fruits and vegetables

ANTIOXIDANTS: Dark chocolate (yep!), black coffee, green tea, fruits, vegetables, whole grains, citrus

FIBER: Fruits, cruciferous vegetables (broccoli, cabbage, cauliflower, bok choy, collard greens, and more), whole grains, seeds (flax, chia, hemp, sunflower), legumes

PROTEIN: Nuts, seeds, poultry, red meats, seafood, dairy, eggs, legumes

HEALTHY FATS: Oils (extra-virgin olive oil, coconut oil), avocados, nuts, seafood, eggs, legumes

Indulgences are those foods that revolve around celebrations, playful moments, and tempting desires, but aren't working for the health of your body. Slide these in here or there but don't make them the focus:

ADDED SUGARS: Refined white sugar, high-fructose corn syrup, molasses

SODIUM: Frozen dinners and pizzas, canned foods that don't say "reduced-sodium" or "no salt added," packaged chips and other savory snacks, salted nuts, salted butter

SATURATED FATS: Processed meats, dairy, butter and margarine, pastries, pies

PROCESSED FOODS: That bag of cookies from your childhood, anything with ingredients foreign to nature (food colorings, preservatives, salts, sugars, gums)

WHOLE FOODS

I talk a lot about the significance of whole foods. I look at food as medicinal, both mentally as a source of comfort, and physically as a source of strength and energy. We all have a responsibility to take care of ourselves, which goes beyond seeing a doctor once a year for a physical. Although Western medicine has saved millions of lives, it's not the only thing that can prevent illness and maintain good health. Food has that power. I use food for the vitality I need to tend to myself, my family, and my job. I also use food to safeguard my children's strength and power their brains so they can reach their full potential. I am very open with my children about the food choices I make for them, specifically why we don't stockpile sugary cookies and fried chips. Cree is deeply knowledgeable about why we don't buy processed foods and understands the impact an abundance of "fun" foods can place on the body. Passing down that sage information has given him the confidence to make healthy choices for himself, too!

Simply put, whole foods—fresh produce, nuts, seeds, proteins, and whole grains—do not undergo extensive processing. Our food industry has run amok, making it challenging to eat clean these days. By utilizing your kitchen instead of eating out or buying packaged meals, you have control of what you and your family are eating. For me, it's all about replacing highly processed foods with whole or minimally processed versions.

A few years back, I followed a very strict diet to reduce inflammation, dodging anything in plastic bags or packaging (both are indications that the food went through some sort of processing) and focusing on fresh, fresh, fresh. However, I have eased up on my restrictions and loosened the rules a little while still adhering to the basic ideas. Because I want to put a meal on the table most nights, I might purchase some packaged items, such as dried herbs and spices, precut vegetables, and canned beans. Still, a few things are always consistent: locally sourced or organic, high-quality proteins, and limited processed foods.

Unfortunately, I waited until I was sick before opening my eyes and taking action. But now I know that to care for my body correctly and sustain well-being, I need to focus on these principles all the time. No shame if you're just starting now! Little steps will guide you to the bigger picture. And for your kids, this book will help introduce flavor. Eventually, hopefully, that will take on a life of its own and spur their curiosity, so you no longer need to wrestle getting veggies into their diet!

Organic

I know this one isn't easy for everyone, but here's something to consider. When produce is grown organically, it is minimally or not at all sprayed with pesticides or herbicides, limiting your exposure to those chemicals. You can scrub or peel the toxins away with many vegetables or fruits, but some chemicals are still absorbed and remain under the peel. Packaged products, such as canned foods or snacks deemed "organic," follow these guidelines and use organic ingredients. I don't want you to overthink this or overreach your budget here, because eating veggies is important either way. If you're going to weave organic into your kitchen, start with the following list. These are the fruits and vegetables sprayed most, and you will see a pattern that the skins are typically thin, making it a homey environment for insects (and chemicals) to dig in. In contrast, something like a banana isn't as vulnerable, hence less spray!

Go organic with these items:

* Apples
* Apricots
* Blueberries
* Celery
* Cherry tomatoes
* Grapes
* Hot peppers
* Leafy greens (spinach, kale, and collards)
* Nectarines
* Peaches
* Potatoes
* Snap peas
* Strawberries (sometimes you can even taste the chemicals!)
* Sweet bell peppers

High-Quality Proteins

I urge you to lean toward meats (beef, chicken, pork, lamb, deli meats) that are organic, grass-fed, antibiotic-free, and have no added hormones. The way our country farms meat these days is less than admirable, and the chemicals used to plump up and keep animals healthy don't just disappear before they're on your plate. Your body takes in the toxins fed to animals. This is why it's best to purchase higher-grade proteins from reputable sources. Look at the packaging to see if it says "no antibiotics" or "no added hormones." Also, try to find proteins (eggs included) that are pasture- or farm-raised, meaning the animals aren't cooped up in deplorable conditions. Instead, they are free to amble and graze on the land. I know it can be a little pricier, but if you make cooking at home a regular habit, you'll save money on restaurant bills, which means wiggle room for quality ingredients. If it's too expensive to go 100 percent high-end proteins, then do a mix! Half of the week full organic, half of the week not.

I chum it up with the butcher as the freshest meats are typically under that glass, and he or she can guide me to the best, most flavorful products available at that time. But ask for farm-raised or grass-fed cuts. If you become besties, they may even give you the bestie cut of the day. Get to know your butcher!

What to look for:

COLOR: Good beef will be vibrantly red in color without signs of gray.

DATE OF PACKAGING: Ensure it's not nearing its end date.

LABELS: No antibiotics and no added hormones are best.

GRASS-FED: Animals fed this way are healthfully nourished and are typically more flavorful than those that are fed corn, wheat, and soy.

FARM-RAISED: Animals that are farm-raised have more space to stretch and move, otherwise they can be cramped and susceptible to disease (hence the use of antibiotics).

Eggs

These days, egg cartons are complicated with their varying labels and language. Yet, once you get the hang of what everything means, you'll know how those ladies live and eat, which makes a difference in the health and flavor of the eggs. My preferences are organic free-range or pasture-raised eggs because I know the feathered gals are well taken care of and live in humane conditions. My biggest advice is to stay away from caged hens that are confined in spaces smaller than a piece of paper. Instead, here are some label terms that I opt for, which I hope will shed some light on how hens are raised and how that impacts the quality of eggs:

CAGE-FREE: These hens are not restricted to cages, but they live in overcrowded buildings. The FDA regulations do not require outdoor playtime for these hens, so many will never feel the warmth of sunshine. If "cage-free" is your only choice on the shelves, grab those instead of the dozen without a designation.

FREE-RANGE: These birds are never confined to cages and are able to access outdoor roaming for up to six hours a day. However, it is not required that these birds feed off living vegetation. Rather, some farmers will sustain their hens with soy and corn, which isn't as healthful but, hey, at least they can stretch.

PASTURE-RAISED: These beauties spread their wings and feed off live vegetation in outdoor pastures. While a dozen of these eggs is typically more expensive, you will notice orange and flavorful yolks that can't be resisted.

Clean Fish

Seafood provides a healthy source of omega-3 fatty acids, which benefits the brain and heart. The American Heart Association recommends eating two servings of fish, a total of eight ounces, a week to get the full health benefit. When purchasing fish, it's important to pay attention to what you're buying and where you are buying from. I seek out seafaring proteins from reputable sources that practice sustainable fishing in locations low in mercury exposure. Ocean sustainability is vital to ensure the fishing practices be done in a way that keeps the ocean's ecosystem intact. On the label, look for "wild-caught" from areas that are not high in water pollution, or "farm-raised" with certifications that specify the fish was farmed responsibly. Monterey Bay Aquarium Seafood Watch, which is an incredible resource for finding quality seafood in your area, has various standards to look for when shopping for farm-raised or wild-caught:

— **CERTIFIED SUSTAINABLE SEAFOOD MSC**
— **BAP**
— **FARMED RESPONSIBLY ASC CERTIFIED**
— **NATURLAND**

You can also utilize companies online that ship direct from fishermen whose sustainable measures adhere to clean farming and quality.

Whole Grains

Whole grains—which include wheat, corn, rice, oats, barley, spelt, rye, and quinoa—are consumed whole, cracked, split, or ground. They provide a big chunk of daily fiber, magnesium, and certain antioxidants that are not derived from vegetables. Look for food labels that say "whole," which means that the end product did not go through significant processing and still retains a lot of nutrients. Today, because consumers find value in whole grains, I don't encounter too much difficulty sourcing whole-grain products. Bleached-flour Wonder bread (a true wonder, indeed) is a thing of yesteryear, and there are whole grains aplenty at the grocery store.

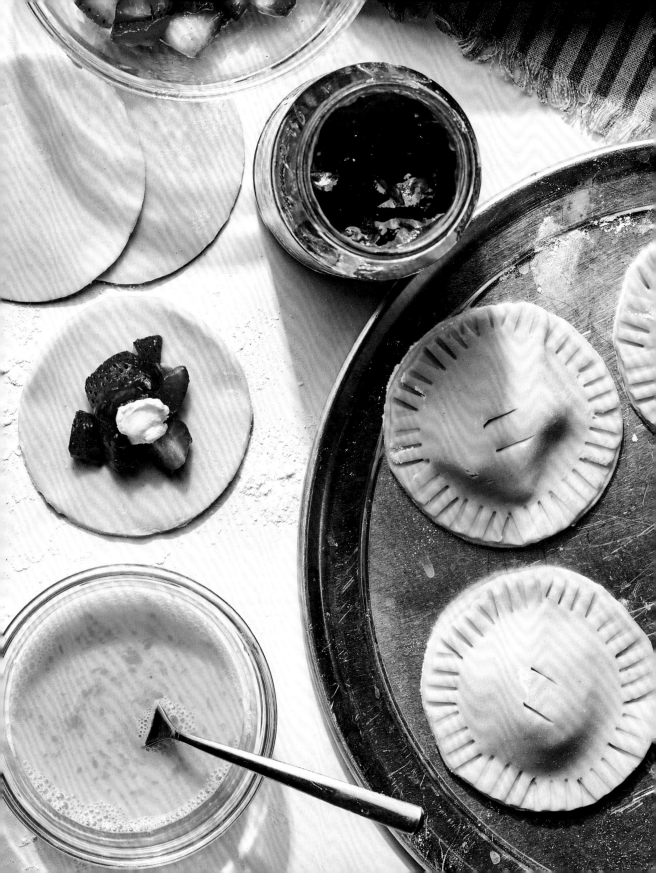

Processed Foods

When we continually eat processed foods, our immune and digestive systems are busy sifting through unnatural ingredients rather than adequately absorbing the needed nutrients. After years and years of this, the body can slowly fall prey to disease. Cutting out processed foods is especially imperative for kids who are growing and developing. I had a pretty rough go eliminating processed, packaged foods when I had to! While I'm on set, cookies and candy are at my disposal and I have to walk by them without diving in, which absolutely breaks my heart! Growing up, I couldn't resist snacking on anything I wanted. All of it was right there for the taking! Eventually, I craved cheese chips more than I did the healthy stuff. When my doctor kicked those vices to the curb, I went through withdrawals. It was crazy, but I adjusted and am better because of it.

I live in a city and do not have access to a full farm in my backyard where I can pick the freshest crop for my daily meals. However, once healthy eating became a habit, I found it pretty easy to locate foods that are not absolute junk. Say, for instance, vibrant fruit snacks made with sugar, high-fructose corn syrup, gelatin, additives, food coloring, flavoring, enhancements, and preservatives. Luckily, this type of fruit snack isn't the only thing on the shelves. I can choose from a multitude of brands made with natural ingredients and real fruit juice instead of dyes and artificial flavoring. I don't mind wandering in an aisle for a while to read nutritional labels. If I don't recognize more than one ingredient on a package, I politely place it back on the shelf and go on my merry way. Those multisyllable tongue twisters are usually additives the body can't properly digest.

Furthermore, just because it says "vegan" doesn't mean it's healthy. Some, not all, of those fake meats are the most processed foods on the market. Imagine the transformation process of vegan chicken nuggets from wheat and corn to something that simulates the look, texture, and flavor of real chicken. Mind you, some vegan alternatives are just fine, but take a gander at the nutritional label before tossing them in your cart.

Added Refined Sugars

Speaking of nutritional labels, if "sugar" or a refined sugar variant is the first ingredient listed, it's probably best to move on to something else. While our body needs some sugar in the form of glucose, it does not need refined sugars (white sugar, high-fructose corn syrup, brown sugar, powdered sugar). In 2020, Ireland's Supreme Court considered bread from Subway "not real bread," according to their standards of what "real bread" should be. Why? Because 10 percent of its weight comes from its sugar content. When I heard this, I was stunned. I know a lot of the sugar we consume is under a guise like this, but that's a heck of a lot of sugar for bread. The New Hampshire Department of Health and Human Services shows that the average American consumes almost 152 pounds of sugar in one year, which comes out to approximately 6 cups per week. That is crazy. Believe it or not, most of our sugar intake is not from confections and other foods we categorize as "sweet." Instead, we are consuming sugars added to everyday foods: canned soups, bread, crackers, bottled beverages, salad dressings, to name only a very few. When looking at a nutritional label, scan down to sugars and next to it you will see the percent and grams of "added sugars." That number indicates the amount of sugar added during processing. Some foods contain natural sugars, but be aware of the added processed sugars.

SEASONAL GUIDE

Buying in-season produce increases the chances of you purchasing freshly harvested products. Take it to the next level and look for "local" to cut back on the time and distance that produce had to travel before it got to you so you could take a bite of it. When fruits are picked and shipped long distance, they are nowhere near ripe because they need to ripen during transport and stocking. Otherwise, they'll end up rotten in the produce section. Getting produce from farms near you means getting produce that is allowed to stay on the tree or in the soil longer, ultimately packing more nutrients and flavor.

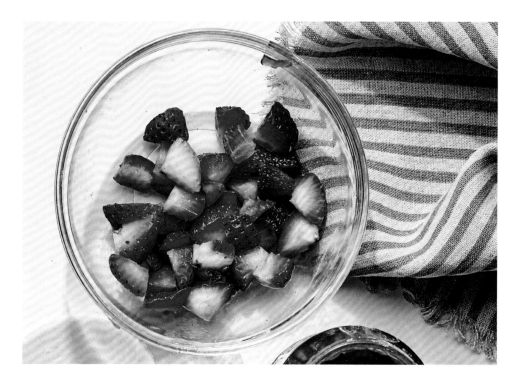

Spring Fruits

- APPLES
- APRICOTS
- BANANAS
- KIWIFRUIT
- LEMONS
- LIMES
- PINEAPPLES
- STRAWBERRIES

Spring Veggies

- ASPARAGUS
- AVOCADOS
- BROCCOLI
- CABBAGE
- CARROTS
- CELERY
- COLLARD GREENS
- GARLIC
- KALE
- LETTUCE
- MUSHROOMS
- ONIONS
- PEAS
- RADISHES
- RHUBARB
- SPINACH
- SWISS CHARD
- TURNIPS

Summer Fruits

- APPLES
- APRICOTS
- AVOCADOS
- BANANAS
- BLACKBERRIES
- BLUEBERRIES
- CANTALOUPE
- CHERRIES
- HONEYDEW MELON
- LEMONS
- LIMES
- MANGOES
- PEACHES
- PLUMS
- RASPBERRIES
- STRAWBERRIES
- TOMATOES
- WATERMELON

Summer Veggies

- BEETS
- BELL PEPPERS
- CARROTS
- CELERY
- CORN
- CUCUMBERS
- EGGPLANT
- GARLIC
- GREEN BEANS
- LIMA BEANS
- OKRA
- SUMMER SQUASH
- TOMATILLOS
- ZUCCHINI

Fall Fruits

- APPLES
- BANANAS
- CRANBERRIES
- GRAPES
- KIWIFRUIT
- LEMONS
- LIMES
- MANGOES
- PEARS
- PINEAPPLES
- RASPBERRIES

Fall Veggies

- BEETS
- BELL PEPPERS
- BROCCOLI
- BRUSSELS SPROUTS
- CABBAGE
- CARROTS
- CAULIFLOWER
- CELERY
- COLLARD GREENS
- GARLIC
- GINGER
- GREEN BEANS
- KALE
- MUSHROOMS
- ONIONS
- PARSNIPS
- PEAS
- POTATOES
- PUMPKIN
- RADISHES
- RUTABAGAS
- SPINACH
- SWEET POTATOES (YAMS)
- SWISS CHARD
- TURNIPS
- WINTER SQUASH

Winter Fruits

- APPLES
- AVOCADOS
- BANANAS
- GRAPEFRUIT
- KIWIFRUIT
- LEMONS
- LIMES
- ORANGES
- PEARS
- PINEAPPLES

Winter Veggies

- BEETS
- BRUSSELS SPROUTS
- CABBAGE
- CARROTS
- CELERY
- COLLARD GREENS
- KALE
- LEEKS
- ONIONS
- PARSNIPS
- POTATOES
- PUMPKIN
- RUTABAGAS
- SWEET POTATOES (YAMS)
- SWISS CHARD
- TURNIPS
- WINTER SQUASH

BALANCING MEALS

As I've previously mentioned, maintaining the fuel in your daily jet-pack can propel you into a productive superhero void of slumps and fatigue. All of our diets differ, so for me, that may mean three meals and two snacks, whereas it can mean something entirely different for you. The thing to consider is what you're eating during your mealtimes and finding balance among them. Let's say I gobble up the cheesy marvels of a breakfast burrito. Later, I know I should probably eat a salad to balance out that whirlwind of eggy extravagance. Otherwise, I'll be dragging my feet all day. These are the things I think about for each meal:

Breakfast

I love breakfast because it jump-starts my day. Knowing that it can supply or deplete my steam are prime factors on my plate or bowl. Some say it's the most important meal of the day, and you better believe I agree with that! When I wake up, the last time I ate was most likely at dinner, potentially 12 to 15 hours prior. The last time I had water? Probably after six to eight hours of sleep (four hours these days, unless I woke up for a sip). At this stage, my internal organs are ready and willing to power my day by metabolizing food into energy. They are amped, and they are THIRSTY. Immediately following dreamland, I drink a full glass of H_2O to wake up my organs. Then I eat breakfast.

My breakfasts are a well-balanced combination of protein, fat, and carbs. Together, that trio is the energizer necessary to awaken and sustain my body for hours. I usually make something quick on the weekdays and ring in weekend morning festivities with something more substantial because we have the time, and it's fun! If mornings are chaotic, there are plenty of options to help lift that burden. Most of the breakfast recipes you'll soon explore can be made in bulk to grab while running out the door.

When I was a kid, I poured myself a bowl of colorful fruit-shaped sugar bombs or cinnamon-coated squares every day. If I had rice cereal, I'd dump sugar all over it because my morning sweet tooth had a lot of power over me. Not anymore! Today, I'm way more conscious of my first meal of the day, with a boost of whole-grain cereals (seven grams of sugar or less) or homemade granola. You know, store-bought often contains more than twenty grams of added sugar in only one-third cup! Sugar spikes insulin, then causes a crash—what goes up, must come down. Dosing with sugar in the morning leads to midmorning slumps. Therefore, I skip breakfast sweets or make reduced-sugar versions at home!

I'm a closet snacker. I love snacks. I love nibbling away at night and throughout the day. Thus, I need to focus on healthier choices, some of which I covered previously, so I'm not habitually devouring junk. Snacks are great if you experience a growling belly or a dip in energy between meals. Again, food is fuel, and by providing the body with premium fuel, you can rev your engine and get that zip you need to keep moving. When I choose snacks, I look closely at the nutritional label to assess sugar content and additives—such as food coloring and words I don't understand—then I consider the processing. I used to eat a bag of cheesy chips and those crunchy onion rings. How does one make an onion ring without any onion? It's a mystery. Think of snacks as the pit stop on a road trip sustaining you until the next fuel station: lunch or dinner!

Lunch

I'm an advocate for a hearty yet light lunch filled with protein, greens, and a carb. In college, a professor told me, "Carbs help your brain focus," and I need that! I consider this meal a substantial pick-me-up that won't weigh me down. Meaning, I choose light sustenance: pasta with veggies and chicken, or a sandwich piled with mixed lettuce and sliced turkey, or a salad tossed with a kaleidoscope of produce.

Kids require a little different construction. My mom worked her butt off to care for and feed us. And back in the day, prepared store-bought lunches were small miracles for working mommies like her. So we had a constant rotation of those, along with sugary juices and PB&Js in our lunch boxes. Side note: I hated when my sandwich slipped to the bottom of my backpack and got smashed from the weight of my apple or orange. A big lunch wrecker, if you ask me. Did that ever happen to you? Ugh, the worst!

Today, I know those premade lunches aren't the best for the body. I prepare lunches in a bento box (a little airtight container with sections similar to those premade lunches) and fill it up with colorful nutrition. I add an assortment of homemade snacks (carrot sticks, dehydrated apple slices, trail mix, bagel poppers) and munchies such as a sandwich or tortilla pinwheels!

Dinner

And of course, the finale: dinner. The time when everyone is home and settling down, ready to reconnect and dig in. By now, we all know my passion for this particular time of day so I won't repeat myself. Okay, fine, I will. I love it so much! It is when I'm at my happiest and when my soul is full and warm. Balance here means getting all the food groups on the plate: carbs, veggie or fruit, and protein. This can come in the form of one heaping spoonful of Chicken Teriyaki Bowl (page 204), a slice of pizza topped with sautéed spinach, or a lean protein paired with veggies and a sweet potato. The USDA has a great program called "MyPlate," where they suggest filling half the plate with veggies, which I love for a couple of reasons. One, it doesn't leave enough room for the more tempting foods and two, I know I'm getting my vitamins, minerals, and fiber. I dedicate the other half of the plate to protein and starch, as you'll see in the indulgence of Meatloaf Cupcakes with Mashed Potato Frosting (page 230), am I right? Yes, I am, just you wait.

BALANCING NEEDS

There are various dietary needs and finicky eaters in today's world, and it may feel like a one-pan meal is out the window. But that's not the case here. Throughout the recipe section, I provide swaps specific to each recipe, but the general rule of thumb is that you don't need to cook different meals for each person in the household. At first, the most challenging part as an evolving mommy was balancing everyone's preferences, but now I ask myself, "What do the kids want, what does Cory want, and what can I eat?" And from there, I whisk up some thoughts. I apply tricks to make well-known dishes easier, such as my one-pot Italian Pot Pie (page 179), or healthier versions of classics, like my family's fave Creamy "Alfredo" Pasta (page 212), where I keep the succulent, silky texture of the "Alfredo," but eliminate the dairy and heavy weight by blending white beans into a velvety sauce, rather than using a bucket of heavy cream. It caters to my health needs and still delights the taste buds of my hubby and kids. In this way, you can balance everyone's wants and needs in the same meal.

I've learned over the years by quick-fixing on my YouTube channel that almost every dish can be flexible. Pancakes made on a sheet pan (see page 128), for example, is a go-to for us that pleases everyone's palate by being easily adaptable. Once I pour the pancake batter into the pan, I add fruit on my portion, dark chocolate chips on Cairo and Cree's, and nothing on Cory's because he prefers good ol'-fashioned pancakes. Three variations on one pan! That also goes for dinners where everyone can construct their own masterworks. During our beloved Baked Potatoes night, I prepare the base and let everyone pick and choose their toppings (see Loaded Potato Bar, page 223). My dad used to do this all the time for tacos, allowing our creativity to conceive the dish we wanted while he made the taco of his dreams. You can do that with a weekly Homemade Pizza Bar (page 238) and Super Nachos with Vegan Cheese Sauce (page 227). Create the base and invite everyone to make the entrée they want!

So, how do you balance the needs of various eaters—whether they are picky, have food sensitivities, or generally can't be bothered with adventure—without preparing separate dishes for each one of them?

Picky Eaters

If you have a picky eater in the household (ahem, a toddler), incorporate them into the process and make them feel like they're a part of choosing, rather than being the outcast who doesn't like what everyone else wants. There are a lot of factors that can go into why someone won't eat something, but for the most part, I've found that fostering positive experiences around food and giving them a choice in what is on their plate can solve that issue. I still have the power, but they'll feel like they have more of a stake in the meal. For kids, I have a few tips:

BRING THEM TO THE STORE WITH YOU. You can kind of manipulate this to balance their needs and that of the rest of the household, but encourage them to pick some of the fruits, veggies, and foods to fill the pantry. If you don't want them to go too wild, just lead them to certain sections and bypass junk and desserts. Allowing them to choose gives them pride and involvement in their food choices.

DEVELOP THEIR RELATIONSHIP TO FOOD. Pair food with fun experiences. That can mean jovial conversations around the table, playfully plating the meal, or getting them involved in the cooking process (more on this later!). Create adventures to make it exciting. Rather than saying, "Here are some carrots, eat them," give it a little PR spin by reframing it: "Look at the carrot torpedoes!"

KIDS AND ADULTS ARE EQUAL. Of course, this depends on the age, but once they're old enough to eat solid foods, serve them what you eat, so they feel like a grown-up. This may not work for everyone, but point it out, "Wow, Cairo, you are such a big girl eating like Mommy, Daddy, and your brother!"

BE SNEAKY. I give this a little more razzle-dazzle on pages 119 to 120, but know there are ways to provide nutrients without giving the undesired ingredient the leading role.

UNDERPROMISE, OVERDELIVER. When Cree was a little cutie toddler, I gave him small portions of the veggies so I didn't overwhelm him. Kids can easily become stressed out if they need

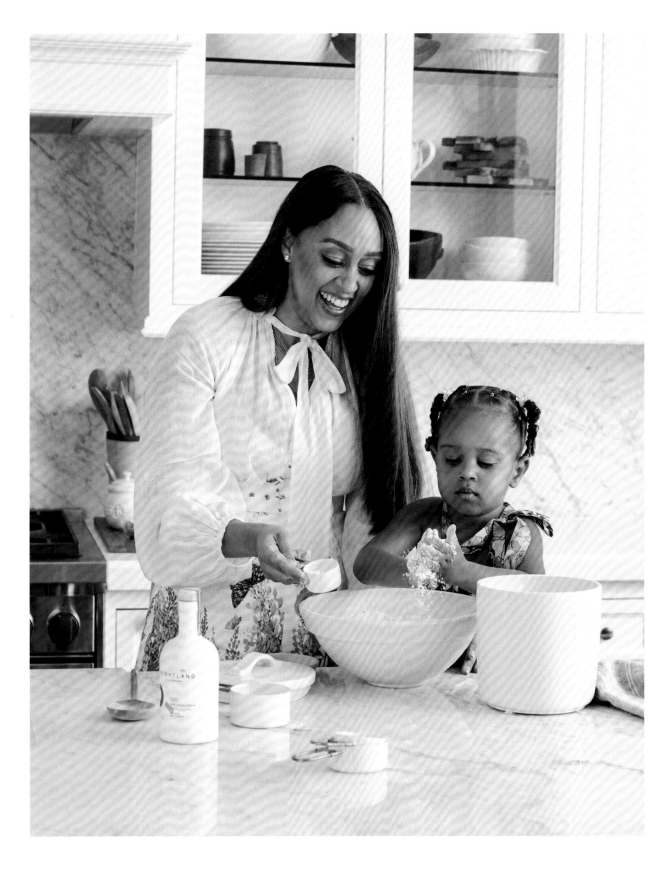

to eat five broccoli florets. I start small, work my way up, and don't force it. They will discover their preferences when they feel they're allowed to make choices rather than being pushed into it.

BE PATIENT. A kid's palate may take longer to develop than an adult's—no need to rush them through the produce aisle to experiment with every fruit or veggie. Work them in slowly and allow him or her to grow into their preferences.

Eaters with Food Sensitivities

If everyone in your house has a different intolerance or sensitivity to a food, then this can become very tricky. But if it's just one person, get them involved. Today, there are so many products to accommodate different allergies or sensitivities. It's easier now than ever to work in food that won't upset their system while sticking to the quick fix schedule. If you're making spaghetti for the entire family but one person is gluten intolerant, use gluten-free noodles. Or, make the fixings for everyone and boil a small batch of the gluten-free stuff to toss with the sauce separately. There are so many alternatives out there, and for *most* things, a swap will work. My suggestion here is to make the bulk of it (or do a swap) and serve the adjusted dish to the eater with the food sensitivity instead of cooking a whole new meal with more pots, pans, and time.

You gotta tiptoe around baked goods, though. The gluten-free flours or nondairy milks don't always do the job like the OGs, so it's best to proceed with caution. I've made a lot of mistakes by trying quick baking swaps. However, I've also made some crowd-pleasers by following specific gluten-free recipes (and some gluten fanatics didn't even realize they were eating something different . . . shhh!).

GENERAL SWAPS AND TIPS

Get cushy, and fashion your own style of recipes! For savory dishes, swaps are flexible and can tend to your needs almost effortlessly. If there's an ingredient you don't particularly fancy, give another one a go. If you can't find kale at the store, spinach or Swiss chard work as good switcheroos. Start with little adjustments, and soon tailoring will become spontaneous!

Baking, on the other hand, is more precise and scientific. Each ingredient serves a specific purpose, and swaps take more tinkering. For instance, the fats in milk and butter leaven. Also, the gluten-free flour for breads doesn't create that same airiness and sponge as all-purpose flour, which binds everything together for that chewy, crunchy goodness we all love about bread. While you can generally adjust for your needs, it may take a little research and trial and error. The following swaps are my go-tos:

ALL-PURPOSE FLOUR

✶ Gluten-free all-purpose flours: **For all baking recipes in this book that call for all-purpose flour, you can replace it with a gluten-free version. I'm not talking almond flour or rice flour, however. Look for blends that specifically work as cup-for-cup replacements for all-purpose.**

REFINED WHITE SUGAR

✶ Coconut sugar, maple syrup, honey, agave

COCOA POWDER

✶ Raw cacao: **"Cocoa" powder is refined and often includes added sugars and dairy, whereas "raw cacao" is pure and packed with antioxidants, magnesium, and iron. Raw cacao is more bitter than regular cocoa powder, but you can balance this by adding sweeteners!**

DAIRY

✶ Sour cream: **Greek yogurt (to lower fat and calories, and also for the added benefit of probiotic bacteria)**

✶ Ricotta: **Cottage cheese (to lower fat and calories)**

✶ Dairy milk: **Coconut milk works well because it contains more fat, but unsweetened nut milk is also fine.**

✶ Cheese: **Nutritional yeast has a nutty flavor that creates a delish vegan cheese, like in my Super Nachos with Vegan Cheese Sauce (page 227).**

BUTTERMILK

✶ Mix 1 cup milk + 1 teaspoon lemon juice or distilled white vinegar and let sit for 15 minutes. You can also use nondairy milk for this swap.

PASTA

* Spiralized zucchini, butternut squash
* Spaghetti squash
* Hearts of palm noodles (the most available brand is Palmini)
* Gluten-free pasta variations: There are plenty to choose from now, including pasta made from lentils, chickpeas, rice, and sweet potatoes!

RICE

* Cauliflower rice, quinoa

POTATOES

* Plantains (for soups/stews)
* Sweet potatoes

MASHED POTATOES

* Cauliflower
* Celery root
* Parsnips
* Turnips

TORTILLAS

* Lettuce leaves
* Cabbage leaves
* Almond flour tortillas
* Thinly sliced jícama

GROUND BEEF

* Turkey
* Chopped mushrooms
* Lentils
* Tofu

PEANUT BUTTER

* Almond, sunflower, pecan, or hazelnut butter

BROTH

* Low-sodium bouillon (powder, cubes, or paste)

MAYONNAISE
(IN RECIPES, NOT ON A SANDWICH)

* Low-fat mayo
* Greek yogurt

SOY SAUCE

* Tamari, liquid aminos

CORNSTARCH (WHEN USED FOR THICKENING A SAUCE)

* Rice flour
* Tapioca starch
* Arrowroot

OLIVE OIL

* Coconut oil
* Ghee

BREAD CRUMBS

* Panko
* Ground nut flours
* Ground oats

FRESH HERBS

* Dried herbs: When you are quick-fixing a meal or if you can't find a fresh herb at the store, you don't need to run around town tracking it down. Dried herbs will almost always do the job when the herb is used for flavoring, but not if it's the base (like for a pesto, herbaceous sauces, or salsas). The general rule: 1 teaspoon of dried herb for every 1 tablespoon of fresh herb.

DEVELOPING YOUR SKILLS

If you're a budding cook, think of this as building a relationship. Usually, you don't get married immediately. You get to know your partner first. You become comfortable. You slowly reveal your vulnerabilities. You make mistakes, and when you do, all is forgiven. Your relationship with the kitchen is similar. Snuggle up and get comfy. If a meal disappoints or if you overcook the roast, then better luck next time! My momma used to say, "Dust yourself off and just try again!" I use that motto daily, especially with any cooking mishaps. It may be the end of a dish, but it's not the end of the world!

In its most basic terms, cooking is combining ingredients and manipulating them (heating, blending, seasoning, chopping, baking, and so forth) to form a dish. Remember, you don't need to be an all-star chef to make a memorable dinner. I genuinely mean that. If you master the basics and ease into cooking with an upbeat attitude, you will fix goodies you never thought possible. Recipes are fundamental step-by-step resources to guide you through your voyage. They're not meant to chain you down but rather teach you flavors and techniques. I am, to this day, still learning new skills and ideas that enthuse my spirit. Aside from showing up with confidence and a playful approach, I believe flexibility is key! Once you've harnessed the basics, home in on the magic of spontaneity.

A good cook is someone who embodies the very act of cooking and instills soul into a dish. Watching my mom cook, I observed her enjoyment, even if smoke started billowing from the oven and a curse word accentuated the moment. Cooking made my mom happy, which made me want to do it, too. Imagine a singer. Mariah. Yes, her. That voice is technically one of the best in the world. Think about her singing "One Sweet Day" in the studio, closing her eyes and waving her hand to express the words. Girl has SOUL. If she just stood there and let words fall out of her mouth into a microphone, I don't think I would've listened to it again. But with her conviction behind it, I had that song on repeat for years. In Italy, I tasted soul in every scoop of gelato or forkful of polenta. In my house, we got soul!

It's okay to feel frustrated if you aren't a whiz right off the bat; cultivating skills takes time and patience. I tap into two things to seize my kitchen prowess: the effective use of a knife and being acquainted with flavor.

Using Your Chef's Knife

The first time I attempted to use a knife accurately, I knew I had a long road ahead of me. I became accustomed to a manic up and down chop method that expedited the process to no one's benefit. Ingredients ended up all over the place, and no wildly chopped piece was similar in size to another, which impacts cooking times. Watching Food Network experts, I saw I had it all wrong and committed to slowing down until I understood the technique. YouTube had just hit the Internet, and I looked for a video on how to cut an onion. In the video, the chef explained gripping the knife and gently swaying the blade through the onion rather than slamming it down. The mechanics felt awkward at first. Every time I wanted to revert to my old ways and rush through the chopping process, I took a breath and slowed down to remember the proper mechanics. Eventually, I worked my way back to speedy slicing, but this time with accuracy and flow.

Using a knife properly will not only help avoid injuries but will also foster proficiency. If you cut, chop, and slice effectively, it makes a difference in efficiency and the ingredient's integrity. For instance, you may have heard a chef use the term "chiffonade" when referring to cutting delicate ribbons from whole basil leaves. Chefs prefer this method because the soft herb is gently cared for rather than being pulverized to shreds. We are not professional chefs here, we are home cooks, and I'm pretty confident no one expects perfectly symmetrical cubes or matchsticks every time. However, the correct use of a knife is a game changer.

There are three main components: the knife itself, the gripping hand, and the assisting hand.

Knife

The knife you use the most should have a blade between 8 and 10 inches in length. There are a lot of great, inexpensive knives out there, but I recommend Wüsthof, as they run the gamut from novice to professional with products in every price range.

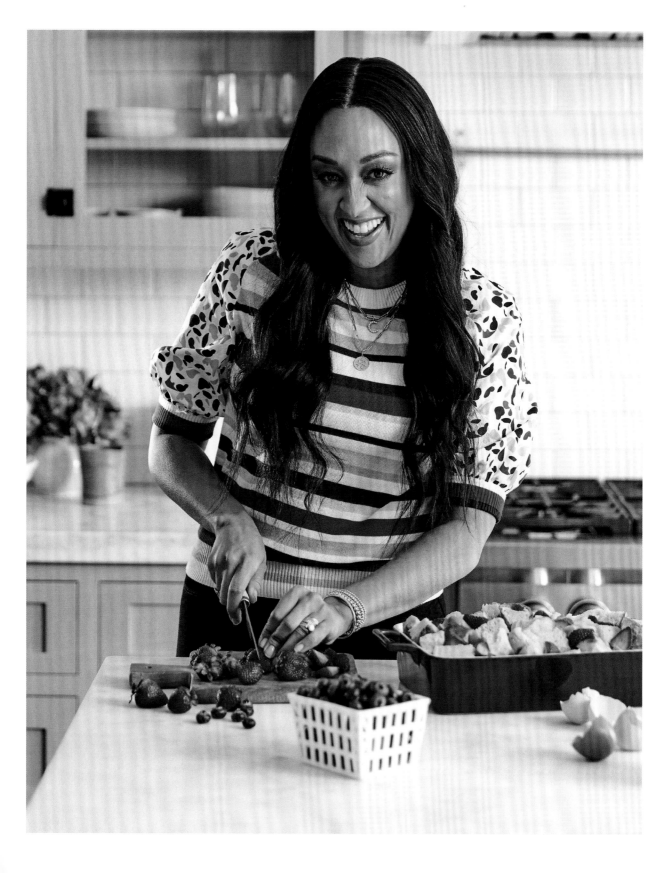

Grip

Hold the handle lightly, avoiding a choke hold. Relax the hand and place your thumb on the blade's bottom where the handle and the blade meet, also known as the "heel." This will help keep a steady yet relaxed grip and give you more stability on the knife.

Assist

You want to use your other hand as a guide on the ingredient, curling your fingers and pressing your top knuckles gently on the ingredient to keep it from moving around the cutting board. Curling your digits protects them. This may feel clumsy at first; in fact, this is the part I struggled with the most, but I took it very slowly until it felt natural. As you cut, chop, and slice, gradually move the assisting hand backward as the knife follows.

Ready, Set, Chop!

Rather than slamming the knife through an ingredient like a guillotine, rock it gently with the easy sway of a rocking chair. Place the knife's tip at the front of the ingredient and rock it down and forward through the ingredient. Sticking to the swaying motion will keep the ingredient from bruising and help you safely make your way through it. The longer the blade, the longer this slide stroke will be, but the size is personal preference.

Caring for Your Knife

Sharpening my knives reminds me of polishing shoes: brand-new again without spending the money on a shiny pair! The blade will be in tip-top shape if you sharpen it before it gets dull, around four times a year. You know a knife has reached that point when you catch yourself sawing a tomato only to find the skin wrinkled and the tomato still whole. A sharp knife will glide through it with grace. You can find sharpening tools online. I prefer the two-stage brands over the honing steel (which looks like a wand) because it is easier for me to handle and sharpen with accuracy. At farmers' markets near me, I see a knife sharpener giving knives the professional touch while his customers shop. Also, check with your local crafts store! They often provide bimonthly sharpening services for fabric scissors and knives.

Washing by hand also preserves the life span of your knives. The heat of the dishwasher can dull the blade and handle.

FLAVOR

Understanding the symphony of flavors will take you from amateur to exceptional, and will help you feel comfortable improvising in the kitchen. The flavor of food is developed when you know how to work with flavor profiles, adding spices and seasonings to emphasize an ingredient's natural blessings. Salt and pepper are in almost every savory recipe I've come across. The S&P power couple is the exclamation point at the end of a sentence, underscoring an ingredient's God-given assets. For the sake of a primer, I'll walk you through my staples with some examples of regional cuisines and their well-known flavors.

Your Spice Rack

Filling up a spice rack can get costly, so know that amassing a big collection isn't necessary. There are only a few that are used frequently in basic cooking. If you want to splurge on saffron, go ahead, but use it to make something great before it loses character on the shelf. Otherwise, stick to the essentials and become acquainted with which ones complement each other. This way, if you're in a bind with nothing to cook, you know your handy spices will have your back to add some pizzazz to a plain tomato sauce or make grilled chicken breasts tastier.

Some spices have a "cooling" effect, whereas others are "warming." In a literal sense, certain ingredients are poised to trigger a sensory response. Cayenne, ginger, and pepper are warming spices that heat the body. You may sweat when eating spicy foods because your body is trying to cool off. Cooling spices, such as cardamom, coriander, and mint, stimulate digestion without causing a personal summer. Here are the staple dried herbs and spices I use on repeat, no matter the season or day of the week:

BAY LEAF: Earthy and slightly floral, this herb adds essence to liquid bases, such as soups and stews. Its aromatics bring delightful back notes to roasts, tagines, and other long-cook methods. You may not initially think bay leaf matters until you take it away, then you try to decipher what's missing.

— Substitute: ¼ teaspoon dried thyme for 1 bay leaf

— Pairs with: Allspice, marjoram, parsley, rosemary, sage, thyme

GROUND CARDAMOM: A little goes a long way and adds fragrant, minty, floral notes to either savory or sweet dishes. If your recipe calls for nutmeg and you don't have any, a tiny pinch of cardamom will do. And for a unique twist to your morning cup of brew or iced coffee, add a dash to the ground coffee before brewing.

— Substitute: Equal parts cinnamon and nutmeg or cinnamon and ginger

— Pairs with: Anise, caraway, cinnamon, citrus, cloves, coriander, cumin, curry, paprika, saffron

CAYENNE: Packs heat without shifting the flavor. This is an easy one to eliminate without impacting the dish too much.

— Substitute: Hot paprika (not smoked), red pepper/chile flakes

CINNAMON: Described as sweet, woodsy, spicy, and hot, cinnamon enhances the flavors of fruits in sweet dishes but adds a warm undertone in savory ones. Also lovely for an indulgent morning of cinnamon toast.

— Substitute: Allspice (but allspice is more robust and can quickly overpower a dish if you add too much)

— Pairs with: Allspice, cardamom, chili powder, cloves, coriander, cumin, fennel, nutmeg, saffron, turmeric

CORIANDER: Produced from the dried seeds of the cilantro plant, it is peppery, earthy, and citrusy.

— Substitute: Caraway seeds, cumin

— Pairs with: Allspice, anise, basil, cardamom, cilantro, cinnamon, citrus, clove, cumin, curry, mint, nutmeg, saffron, turmeric

CUMIN: Very assertive, so it can dominate a dish if overused, but it can also perfectly accent one if used just right. It is a prime ingredient in chili and curry powders and is warm, peppery, lemony, and earthy.

— Substitute: Coriander (they are both seeds from plants in the parsley family)

— Pairs with: Allspice, anise, bay leaf, cardamom, cayenne, chili powder, cinnamon, cloves, coriander, curry, fennel, nutmeg, oregano, paprika, saffron, thyme, turmeric

GARLIC POWDER: As pungent as the real deal and works well when you don't want to fuss with the fresh stuff.

OREGANO: A member of the mint family with an earthier flavor profile, it is used in cuisines across the globe, packs a punch, and provides a great aroma to a dish.

— Substitute: Marjoram or thyme (another member of the mint family)

— Pairs with: Basil, chili powder, chives, cumin, marjoram, mint, paprika, parsley, rosemary, sage, thyme

PAPRIKA: Synonymous with Hungarian and Spanish cuisine, this spice (regular, not smoked) is made from ground and dried sweet peppers, bringing the red pepper notes to dishes that need it without an added heat wave.

— Substitute: Cayenne, chili powder, red pepper flakes (just a little less than the recipe calls for)

— Pairs with: Allspice, caraway, cardamom, curry, garlic, ginger, marjoram, oregano, parsley, rosemary, saffron, thyme, turmeric

PEPPERCORNS: I recommend whole peppercorns and a pepper grinder; freshly grinding releases the pepper flavors at their peak.

SEA SALT: Salt is to food what the fairy godmother is to Cinderella; it illuminates the beauty already there and brings out the aura that is hidden behind the curtains. I recommend sea salt because it is less refined.

THYME: Its subtlety brings a bright, earthy essence to a dish without taking center stage. Rubbing fresh thyme into your hand releases a soft lemony fragrance that is just lovely.

— Substitute: Oregano and marjoram (they're all related!)

— Pairs with: Allspice, basil, bay leaf, chive, clove, coriander, curry, dill, fennel, lavender, marjoram, mint, nutmeg, oregano, paprika, parsley, rosemary, sage

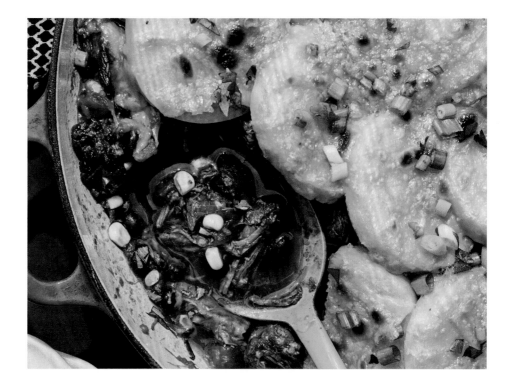

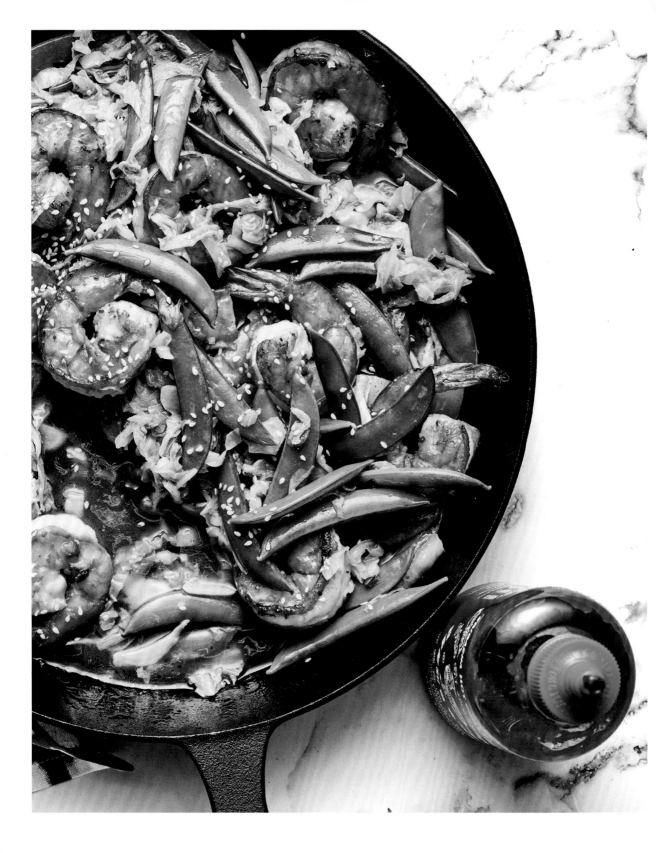

REGIONAL NUANCES

Food brings identity to people around the world and illuminates our good earth's riches. Agriculture is the most significant influence that shapes global cuisine. It fosters the plants that feed the animals and the animals and plants that feed us. When looking at regional dishes, you will see that ingredients are fruits of the land impacted by the climate.

Across the globe are hallmark foods that embody cultures. What is passed down from generation to generation defines dishes, menus, and traditions specific to that country. In Mexico, a Yucatán village still cooks indigenous Mayan cuisine, eagerly trying to inspire their kin to grasp these ancient techniques that distinguish them. In Italy, families work around a kitchen table shaping gnocchi and telling stories, grandchild learning from grandmother as she flicks those little potato dumplings from the back of the fork onto the table where the others are piled up. In Japan, the tea ceremony is a sacred Buddhist tradition, meant to marry harmony, respect, purity, and serenity. Every country—and every region within that country—has interpretations handed down and influenced by its available resources. Here in America, you'll find fry bread in New Mexico that nods to a

time-honored provision of the Navajo Nation, clambakes in the Northeast to celebrate the seasonal Atlantic catch, or barbecue in the South that honors community.

Once you learn the flavors of countries and regions worldwide, you will look inside your pantry and instinctively know what pairs best. I've loved playing with these flavors in my own cooking, some of which inspired dishes within this cookbook!

Following is a list of herbs and spices synonymous with different countries; those scrumptious affinities that pay homage to the land.

CARIBBEAN: My mom's side is from the Caribbean, and I grew up surrounded by dishes layered in bright, citrusy, upbeat flavors. Due to its location, Caribbean food is a fusion emblematic of its indigenous people and centuries of global explorers from Africa, Europe, India, and China. One prominent spice that defines stews, braises, and desserts is cinnamon. It is everywhere!

Allspice, bay leaf, chile peppers, cilantro, cinnamon, cloves, curry, dill, garlic, ginger, jerk seasoning, lime, nutmeg, oregano, parsley, tamarind, thyme

CHINESE: After immigrating here, people adapted their recipes to cater to American palates and accessibility of ingredients. Therefore, if you visit China, you may not find Beef and Broccoli or General Tso's Chicken. Instead, you'll see sizzling hot pots, dim sum, and spicy mapo tofu, to highlight just a tiny dot on the spectrum. However, I do find the Chinese-influenced dishes most familiar in our country are the simplest to make at home, some of which you will find in this very book. Considering the country's size, the climate ranges from tropical to subarctic and everything in between, while the land spans mountains, deserts, forests, and rivers. Each region has very distinct accessible resources and thousands of years of tradition as inspiration for the individual regional cuisines. The overarching profile is, however, heartwarming, satiating, and comforting.

Chile peppers, cinnamon, garlic, ginger, hoisin sauce, rice vinegar, scallions, sesame (oil and seeds), soy sauce, star anise, sugar

GREEK: Greece includes landlocked regions, islands, and sea coasts. Traveling from island to island, you'll taste local crops influenced by the weather. Dry landscapes are the result of high winds, and more lush areas are subject to constant rain. Because of this, you may find root vegetables and their greens highlighted across menus, animals flavored from grazing on herbs, or cheeses uniquely flavored from oregano-grazing sheep. However, no matter where you travel, the underlying notes are consistent throughout.

Allspice, anise, basil, bay leaf, cinnamon, cloves, dill, fennel, garlic, honey, mint, nutmeg, oregano, parsley, thyme

ITALIAN: No matter where you go in the world, an Italian restaurant awaits, full of happy diners twirling strands of noodles and jubilantly sloshing glasses of wine. Some of the globe's best-known dishes come from Italy, with climates varying from tropical in the south to frigid in the north. Throughout the landscape, people harvest wheat for pasta, corn for polenta, and rice for risotto, whereas the trees yield olives for oil and plants yield grapes and tomatoes in abundance. Citrus is prominent in the south and brightens its seafood catch. Like other countries, each region takes on its own personality, adapting dishes based on its specific landscape. Yet one thing remains constant: the herbaceous sensibility that brings each dish to life.

Basil, fennel, garlic, lemon, oregano, parsley, red pepper/chile flakes, rosemary, saffron, sage, thyme

JAPANESE: Known for emphasizing each ingredient as naturally and cleanly as possible; you won't find too many spices influencing flavor. Rather, Japanese cooking illuminates purity and quality. Take sushi, for instance. It is fish at its (almost) purest form. Fresh from the ocean, delicately sliced, and so meticulously crafted. Some chefs spend years learning to make sushi rice and only sushi rice before taking the next step in sushi making.

Chile peppers, dashi (a stock made from kelp), ginger, mirin, ponzu sauce, scallions, sesame, wasabi, yuzu

MEXICAN: Due to the country's geographical diversity, you'll see ingredients that range from tropical fruits, wild mountainous game, vibrantly colored corn, beans, squash, tomatoes, and a potpourri of warm and cool spices. If you explore Mexican food beyond tacos and burritos, bright, luscious, earthy dishes deep in flavor will emerge. Oaxaca, for instance, is known for its moles—a sauce made of tomatoes, pumpkin seeds, chile peppers, and chocolate—that vary in color and heat level; tamales wrapped in banana leaves; elote (corn slathered with cream, spices, and lime); and much, much more.

Chile peppers, cilantro, cinnamon, cumin, garlic, lemon, lime, onion, oregano, saffron

SPANISH: Throughout its history, Spain underwent invasion after invasion, with a constant flow of other countries settling in and leaving their mark, both culturally and gastronomically. It is said that Greeks introduced olive oil and the Moors brought saffron, which is present in many of Spain's rice dishes (I'm looking at you, paella!). Otherwise, for inspiration Spaniards reach out to their diverse terrain, sprawling from coast to coast, through mountain ranges, pastures, woods, and farmland. The result is a cuisine filled with seafood, fresh herbs, rice, ham, and spice.

Bay leaves, garlic, lemon, onion, orange, parsley, peppers, saffron, sherry, sherry vinegar, thyme, vanilla

THAI: Spice! I went to a restaurant once and they asked, "On a scale of one to ten, what spice range would you like?" I bashfully said four, as the waitress hesitantly confirmed my choice. Four seemed reasonably low on the scale, but that first bite sure was a smack of heat-scale reality! My lips tingled, sweat beaded on my forehead, and a swift adrenaline rush coursed through my body. Chile peppers are plentiful in Thai cuisine, along with green herbs and vegetation that bring a playground of flavor to the mouth.

Basil, chile peppers, cilantro, coriander, cumin, curry pastes, fish sauce, ginger, lemongrass, lime, mint, sugar, turmeric

PREPARED KITCHEN

prepared ✦ adjective
\ pri-'perd \
made ready for use

Over the years, I've learned that a schedule and lists diminish the possibility of becoming overwhelmed. I'm not fanatical about them, but they keep me on the straight and narrow. *Bam,* watch out, I got my list, and I know where it's taking me. Due to the constant rotation of activities in my life and that of my family, planning helps me manage without going bonkers. Every week I look at my calendar to regroup my mind, body, and spirit, then I plan! Once I sort out my meals and grocery list, I hop in the car, load up on groceries, come home, and organize. This state of preparedness leads me on a path to tasty success.

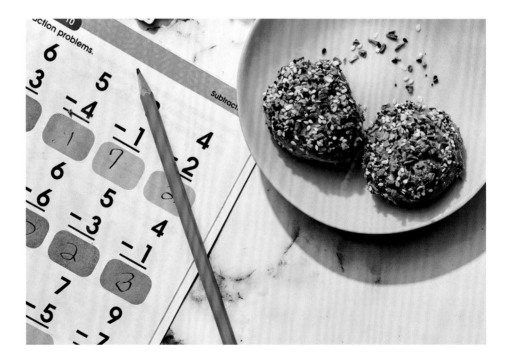

MEAL PLANNING

There's an old Zen saying, "You should sit in meditation for 20 minutes a day. Unless you're too busy, then you should sit for an hour." I feel that way about setting aside time to plan and prepare dinners. When I notice I'm getting swept away, I put in extra time to recenter. I get caught up in my day-to-day hustle a lot, but my upbringing in the kitchen taught me the importance of being present. No better place to be present than the kitchen, am I right? The burgers need to be flipped this second, not whenever I get around to it!

To help persevere in the now, my recipes don't involve hours of prep or drown you in a sea of convoluted steps. That's not how I cook. I keep it basic. The workings of your own home may differ slightly, but the cooking process should be seamless and invigorating. Rally the troops! Assign chores and get the band together for a concert of food. Scheduling and meal prep—paired with family—help all of us ease into the week.

Here's how I do it: I close my eyes and picture myself jamming in Barbados with Rihanna. I get my steps and rhythm down, and I do not stop the music! In fact, I turn it up and sway through the kitchen.

SCHEDULE

I meal plan and hit the grocery aisles every Sunday. At first, this didn't come naturally; I needed to put it on the calendar to hold myself accountable. But now it's a habit. When I wake up on Sundays, I'm thinking about food for the week ahead. I'm a planner with a list. Try to pick a time to sit down and pencil meal ideas. I like to do this in the morning while sipping a cup of coffee. Usually, Cory and the kids are nearby eating at the table with me or running around with fresh energy. Since they're close, I can ask if they'd like anything in particular, which helps with my thought process. When I finish my lists, I head to the store. I do this every Sunday, like clockwork. Schedule; check!

MEAL PLAN

A meal plan cuts out the "Uh-oh! What's for dinner?!" conundrum at 5:00 P.M. on a Thursday when I'm tuckered out. Using a chalkboard, blank calendar, the back of an envelope sitting in the junk mail pile, or your phone's notepad app, brainstorm dinner ideas. I start with the fun meals and balance in the wholesome ones. I focus on more healthful choices during the week and save the fun stuff for the weekend. After a decadent banquet, I want to take a nap! I can't do this Monday through Thursday, but you better believe I snooze on Saturday or Sunday after some comfort food.

Include your family in this task. Huddle up and see what everyone's craving or if there's anything someone wants to learn how to make. Like Taco Tuesdays as a kid. Every week, we warmed the hard shells in the oven to get them buttery and crispy, clamored over the toppings Dad laid out on the counter, and filled them the way we loved. It didn't dawn on me until later in life that Taco Tuesday was a kitchen hack my parents used to cater to everyone's preferences. Now when I sit down to plan the week, I designate one dinner for Cree. Often, it ends up being the pizza bar, but when he fills in that one blank, it's one less slot for me to handle, and I know he will be pumped to lead the program that night!

Once you get your footing, you can incorporate breakfast, lunch, and snacks. If your family loves granola, but you want to cut back on the household's sugar intake, make a batch of Chocolate Cherry Granola (page 143) at the beginning of the week (or double up on the recipe to have more on hand) and feed your family for days. Otherwise, do grab-and-go bites like the Milk & Cereal Bars "On the Go" (page 149) you can snag from the freezer before heading out. The trick here is prepping in advance for a quick fix later. Meal plan, check!

Things to Consider

Meal planning is straightforward, but a few details influence what and why you're cooking. Think about why. Is it to feed the family, or are you feeling adventurous and want to try something new? Have you been craving Grandma's greens, or do you need to fortify someone for a big race or soccer game? The whys can narrow down the galaxy of ideas swirling around the kitchen universe and pinpoint which direction to go.

Read The Room

I believe one of the greatest cooking skills is reading the room: considering the needs of everyone and the surrounding factors that can enhance the enjoyment of a meal. Ask a few questions: "Who are these people I'm cooking for and what do they like?" and "What's the weather for the week?" If the forecast predicts a scorcher, perhaps a soup isn't fitting; instead, chop up a salad and toss it with some of the roasted chicken you plan to make on Sunday night.

Budget

If you want to save on the grocery bill, make it a veggie-heavy week. Produce isn't typically the thing that skyrockets the total on the receipt, it's the protein. Assess your budget and weigh your options. Budget-friendly meals can be composed of the goods in your pantry! Select dishes that call for dried spices and whole grains already in your supply, and shop for inexpensive necessities.

Balance

I'm a huge fan of all things in moderation, and in this case, that means weaving some indulgences into the nutritional mix. Balance here is not leaning on decadent foods, because over time they will bog you down rather than fill you up with nutrients. As mentioned, Monday through Thursday, I'm eating healthy. On the weekend, I'll get down and chow down.

Season

Find the seasonal guides on pages 62 to 64. You'll be hard-pressed to cook a peach tart in the frost of winter. Get familiar with seasonal products and cook in season. This will eventually come easily for you, or perhaps it's already well instilled.

Leftovers

When I meal plan, I always slot in leftovers, which gives me a few days off in the kitchen. Instead of planning for and cooking seven dinners, do three or four, carrying one night's meal to the next. If I were to cook a unique recipe for every meal of the week, that would be twenty-one different recipes to prep, chop, cook, and clean. That's just never going to happen. I cook in batches and my family is happy! Doubling up recipes lets you relax. Dining out or ordering in now and then does, too!

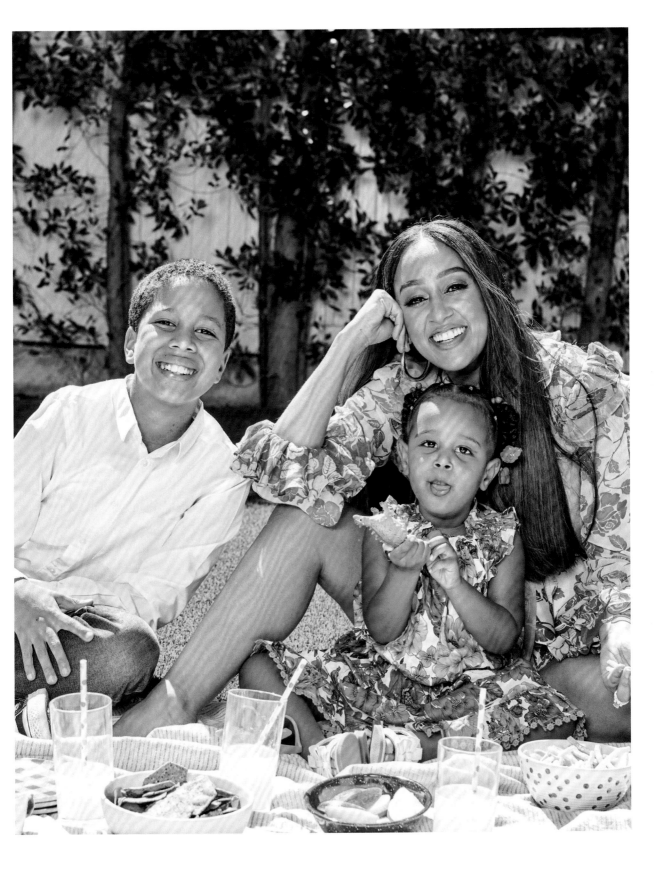

SAMPLE MEAL PLANS

Here are three consecutive sample weeks that account for cooking and leftover days—all the while offering variety. Keep time, nutrition, and balance in mind. I start cooking with Sunday dinner and build upon that, including one homemade snack I make in bulk that I weave in with store-bought ones throughout the week. For these samples, I am not including lunch as that depends on school and work schedules.

WEEK 1

	SUNDAY	MONDAY	TUESDAY	WEDNESDAY	THURSDAY	FRIDAY	SATURDAY
Breakfast	EAT OUT!	Old-School Granola Bars (page 152)	Milk & Cereal Bars "On the Go" (page 149)	Chocolate Cherry Granola (page 143)	*Leftover* Milk & Cereal Bars "On the Go"	*Leftover* Old-School Granola Bars	Baked French Toast (page 134)
Dinner	Chicken Tortilla Soup (page 181)	*Leftover* Chicken Tortilla Soup	Honey-Mustard Salmon with Asparagus & Butternut Squash (page 186)	Spatchcocked Lemon-Herb Chicken with Roasted Baby Potatoes (page 198)	*Leftover* Spatchcocked Lemon-Herb Chicken with Roasted Baby Potatoes with roasted broccoli	Cree's Pick: Homemade Pizza Bar (page 238)!	EAT OUT!
Snack	Trail Mix Bark (page 163) with fruits and veggies (carrot sticks, red peppers, cucumbers and apples)						

	SUNDAY	MONDAY	TUESDAY	WEDNESDAY	THURSDAY	FRIDAY	SATURDAY
✴ **Breakfast**	*Leftover* Baked French Toast	Baked Oatmeal Muffins (page 133)	*Leftover* Baked Oatmeal Muffins	Ham & Cheese Puffs (page 131)	*Leftover* Ham & Cheese Puffs	Oats with fresh fruit	Sheet PanCakes (page 128)
✴ **Dinner**	Creamy Mac & Cheese (page 175)	Chicken Fajita Tacos (page 189)	Beef, Broccoli & Rice (page 192)	*Leftover* Chicken Fajita Tacos	*Leftover* Beef, Broccoli & Rice	Pasta tossed with cheese and butter	**MOVIE NIGHT— ORDER IN!**
✴ **Snack**	Chocolate Chip Protein Bites (page 155)						

	SUNDAY	MONDAY	TUESDAY	WEDNESDAY	THURSDAY	FRIDAY	SATURDAY
✴ **Breakfast**	Cree's Pick: Breakfast Pizza, Two Ways (page 144)	Blueberry Lemon Muffins (page 140)	Cereal	*Leftover* Blueberry Lemon Muffins	Frittata in a Cup (page 147)	Cereal	No-Yeast Cinnamon Rolls (page 257)
✴ **Dinner**	3-Ingredient Roasted Chicken (page 207)	Chicken Teriyaki Bowl (page 204), made with *leftover* 3-Ingredient Roasted Chicken	*Leftover* Chicken Teriyaki Bowl	**ORDER IN!**	Creamy "Alfredo" Pasta (page 212)	Loaded Potato Bar (page 223)	**EAT OUT!**
✴ **Snack**	Old-School Granola Bars (page 152)						

GROCERY LIST

Mom's grocery lists were inventories of the staples: grains, canned veggies, pasta, Spam (yes, you read that right—growing up in Hawaii, Spam was a pantry staple!). I had a blast helping her with the grocery list, and shopping with her cultivated my love for the grocery store. I find a stroll through the aisles incredibly serene; it's a bit of me time to roam through the bounty. Crafting a grocery list keeps me on track during that stroll and saves time (and money!) at the store.

Like Mom, I know the inventory of my kitchen; it lives in my heart! My list is very tailored to my family, but I always start with the ingredients required by my meal plan, then move onto snacks, and so forth. When I start jotting down my list, I group items according to sections to avoid zigzagging. If I write "carrots" between pasta and beans, I may not see it until I've already left the produce aisle. Then I'm forced to go back and forth, which is excellent for reaching 10,000 steps, but not so great on the clock. I also buy only the perishables I know I will use, which prevents food waste and extra spending.

When I'm at the store, I stick to the list and avoid shopping while hungry (if my stomach is growling, I want to buy everything in sight!). I stay on course and veer away from the aisles of wants. You can dodge overspending by keeping your eye on that list!

SAMPLE GROCERY LIST

Here's what a typical weekly list looks like. For the purpose of this book, I included all ingredients necessary for Week 1 meals and snacks, but in italics are the essentials I always have in my kitchen. This will show you how much you already have on hand, and what you need week-to-week are the perishables: fresh produce, dairy, and meats. You'll notice I categorize the list based on sections of the store so I don't find myself rambling back and forth.

Produce

* 1 pound strawberries
* 12 ounces blueberries
* 4 red bell peppers
* 1 small yellow onion
* 1 bunch asparagus
* 2 pounds butternut squash (or 24 ounces precut)
* 3 lemons
* 2 heads broccoli
* 1 bulb garlic
* 2 pounds baby potatoes
* 1 bunch fresh parsley
* 1 bunch cilantro
* 1 package carrots
* 2 English cucumbers
* 2 apples
* 2 avocados
* 1 bulb fennel

Spices

* *Cacao powder*
* *Cinnamon*
* *Vanilla extract*
* *Oregano*
* *Garlic powder*
* *Chili powder*
* *Cumin*
* *Onion powder*
* Fresh cilantro

Canned /Dried Goods

* 32-ounce jar marinara sauce
* 14.5-ounce can diced tomatoes
* 15-ounce can white beans
* 4-ounce bag dried cherries
* 4-ounce bag dried cranberries
* 8-ounce bag raw sliced almonds
* 16 ounces assorted unsalted raw nuts
* (5.5 cups) 32-ounce rolled oats
* 3 cups All-purpose flour
* 8 ounces shredded coconut
* Unsweetened coconut flakes
* 4 ounces shelled sunflower seeds
* 1 bag semisweet chocolate chips

Meat & Fish

* 1 pound boneless, skinless chicken breasts
* 4 (4-ounce) Atlantic salmon fillets
* Whole chicken (3 to 5 pounds)
* Pepperoni
* Ground sausage

Dairy

* 32 ounces Greek yogurt
* 1 dozen eggs
* 32 ounces milk
* Unsalted butter
* Sour cream
* Grated parmesan
* Mozzarella
* 4 ounces Shredded cheddar

Pantry

* Cannellini beans
* ½ cup coconut oil
* Nonstick cooking spray
* Extra-virgin olive oil
* 8-ounce honey
* 1 cup nut butter
* 32 ounces chicken stock
* Tomato paste
* Dijon or whole grain mustard
* Olives
* Caramelized onions
* Jelly/jam
* Maple syrup
* Tortilla chips
* Baking soda
* Baking powder
* Kosher salt
* Black pepper

Grains

* Favorite cereal
* Granola
* 1 loaf bread

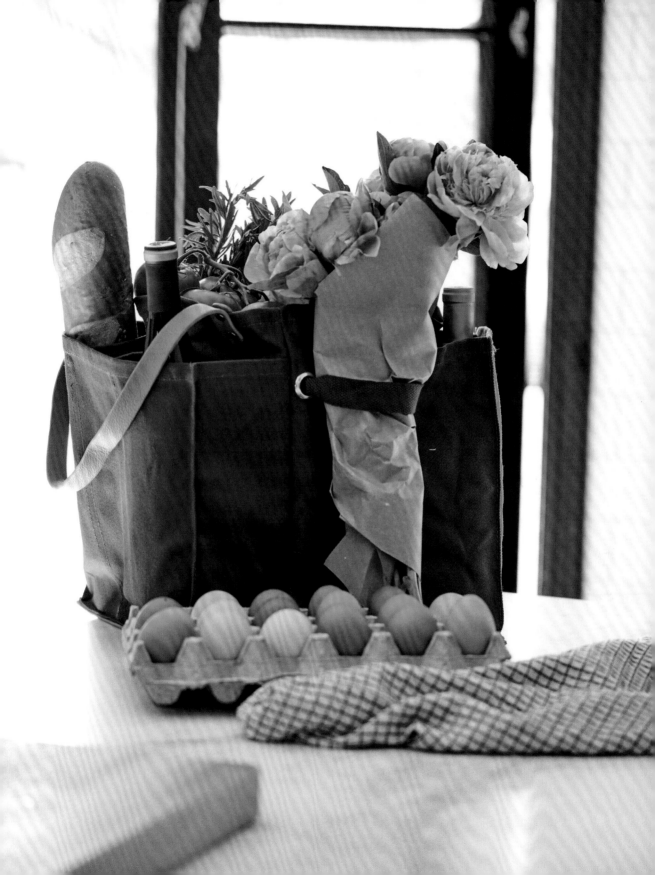

MEAL PREPPING

Realistically, most of the active cooking time is spent prepping: washing, cutting, and measuring. When a busy week is on the horizon, I plan ahead. I achieve a lot after going to the store by cleaning, breaking down, and cutting produce, then storing everything to quickly grab what I need when I need it. This does not have to take all day, and if you can dedicate only 30 minutes to prepping, you'll be surprised how much you can accomplish. No need to overwhelm, but I find laying down this groundwork helps tremendously!

Preparing & Storing Produce

I fill my sink with room-temperature water and give my fruits, veggies, and fresh herbs a quick bath while unloading the rest of the groceries. Any dirt adhering to the food will sink to the bottom, leaving crevasses and leaves clean as a whistle. If you notice a lot of dirt, go for a second round! I air-dry them on a kitchen towel before either chopping or putting in the fridge.

LEAFY GREENS AND HERBS: Bathe, shake off excess water, pat dry with a paper towel, wrap loosely in the same paper towel (the light dampness will help preserve crispness), and put in a reusable produce or plastic zip-top bag. I keep the bag open but roll it to let out excess air. This method maintains freshness longer.

FRUITS AND VEGGIES: Remove from the bag they came home in (the exception here is precut veggies or salad mixes), bathe, lightly scrub, and air-dry. Store on the countertop or fridge. Certain produce thrives in an environment well-suited for them. Tomatoes, for instance, are better off at room temp. Some fruits and veggies release ethylene gas as they ripen, which speeds up ripening for other items around them. Keep these guys to themselves: apples, Asian pears, avocados, bananas, melons, onions, pears, and stone fruits. *Tip: You can take advantage of these gas-emitters if you need something to ripen ASAP, like an avocado. Put it in a paper bag with a banana, close it up, and store at room temperature. The interaction will result in a ripe avocado one or two days faster.*

Fridge vs. Countertop

Oxygen stimulates the production of ethylene gases. If produce were stored in zero-oxygen tanks, it could last more than a year without going bad. There's an apple farm in Sweden that does this, but since we are not a high-tech farm and have only the means of our counter and refrigerator, we must make do.

In most cases, you can judge what goes where by observing its placement in the supermarket. If you grab carrots from the shelves where they are spritzed with that mist of water, you can assume they should go in the refrigerator when you get home. You can leave spuds, onions, and garlic on the counter. If you notice countertop produce ripening faster than expected, go ahead and put them in the fridge! Here's a breakdown.

COOL DARK PLACE

- Garlic
- Onions
- Potatoes
- Sweet potatoes
- Winter squash
  (like butternut and acorn)

COUNTER

- Bananas
- Persimmons
- Pomegranates
- Tomatoes

RIPEN ON THE COUNTER, THEN MOVE TO THE FRIDGE

- Avocado
- Kiwi
- Mango
- Melons
  (honeydew, cantaloupe)
- Stone fruits (plums, peaches, nectarines)

* Apples
* Artichokes
* Asparagus
* Beets
* Berries
* Bok choy
* Broccoli
* Brussels sprouts
* Cabbage
* Carrots
* Celery
* Chard
* Citrus
* Collard greens
* Corn
* Cucumbers
* Eggplant

* Fennel
* Figs
* Ginger
* Grapes
* Leafy greens
  (lettuce, spinach, kale)
* Leeks
* Mushrooms
* Pears
* Peas
* Peppers
* Radishes
* Scallions
* Summer squash
  (zucchini, yellow squash)
* Turnips

Cutting

Trust me on this one, if you cut everything in one fell swoop, you will thank yourself later. If you don't already buy things cut for you (no shame here), chop what you need for the week. A few things I almost always do:

* Peel and cut carrots for snacks
* Break down broccoli and cauliflower so the florets are ready for me
* Trim leaves from beets, fennel, and radishes. Rinse and store the leaves if you want to use them!
* Stem kale, chard, and other sturdy greens. Rinse and chop the leaves, store in a zip-top bag with a paper towel.
* Give zucchini and yellow squash a bath, but wait to chop these. They leak moisture and will ripen quickly.

Waste Not

You may have noticed the term "root to stem" has sprouted recently. Chefs use every part of a vegetable to prevent copious waste. I love this idea and created a little list of various vegetable leaves and stems that you can cook rather than toss.

BEET GREENS: The leaves of beets have the same texture and cooking method as Swiss chard and kale. Give them a good rinse, cut off the stems (see Leafy Green Stems/Ribs, below), chop the leaves, and cook as you would chard or kale.

BROCCOLI STALKS: No need to ignore these regularly overlooked ends. When roasted, they taste like potatoes; when shredded into a slaw, they add character and crunch; and when sautéed and tossed with olive oil, they're firm and lovely.

CELERY LEAVES: If you've never eaten celery leaves, you are in for a treat. These often-tossed delights are spicy and intensely flavorful. Roughly chop for green salads, chicken or egg salads, or soups. They also add quite the kick to fresh juices.

FENNEL FRONDS: I find the fronds aren't overpowering and you can use them as a frolicky garnish, blended into a pesto, or mixed into salads for a very subtle hint of licorice.

LEAFY GREEN STEMS/RIBS: Normally, after stemming and taking the midribs out of kale or chard, these pieces end up in the trash bin. But they can be chopped and sautéed, pickled, or added to soups. Rainbow chard and beet green stems/midribs are bright pink and will change the color of a dish. If that doesn't suit you, lob them into a juicer and watch as the elixir morphs into a lustrous magenta.

RADISH GREENS: These little leaves give oomph to a pesto. They have a fuzzy texture, so I prefer breaking them down in blended recipes instead of eating them whole.

WINTER SQUASH SEEDS: Roasting pumpkin seeds is an annual tradition in my house after carving pumpkins. You can do the same with seeds from other winter squashes, too, and nibble as a snack like you would pumpkin seeds.

Proteins

When I have a hectic schedule ahead, I cook all the proteins one evening and reheat as needed, leaving myself the simple task of preparing just the side dishes. And if I have really prepped ahead of time, then I can cook already chopped veggies on a baking sheet with no stress.

Occasionally I'll buy a whole rotisserie chicken, which is an amazing and versatile ingredient. Generally, though, I make my own, because store-bought rotisserie chickens aren't always farm-raised. The meat from one roasted chicken can be used in a salad on Monday and fajitas on Wednesday. Later on, you'll learn my favorite roasted chicken recipe and three uses throughout the week. I cook ground meats—a great canvas for flavor—at the beginning of the week. If I'm using it for multiple dishes, I season it upon reheating with herbs and spices for tacos, tomato sauce, salad toppers, and so much more.

COOKING IN BULK AND FREEZING

Many recipes in this book are easy to double, even triple, for your leftover needs or to freeze for the weeks ahead. This is incredibly helpful during particularly challenging weeks, like if you've come down with the flu or just had family visit. Knowing I have a frozen meal at the ready keeps me primed for anything.

Before freezing, bring the hot food down to room temperature then pack, seal, and plop it in the icebox. Food safety recommendations advise against letting the food sit out for more than 2 hours, so try not to forget about it while you're in the other room watching and singing to both Trolls movies. And *do not* freeze leftover stews, soup, and stocks in glass containers. The liquid will expand and shatter the glass.

QUICK FIXES

In life, shortcuts get a bad rap. But in the kitchen, I snag each one that comes my way and tuck it into my back pocket. Putting food on the table doesn't need to be a long, drawn-out effort. Welcome a shortcut when you find one and allow for it to be your guiding light. Whatever you can do to fix the food you need, embrace it, hold it near and dear, and run with it . . . all the way into the sunset!

Precut Veggies

My favorite? I. Love. Precut. Veggies. There is no shame in this game. Nowadays, produce sections are packed with a variety of options to reduce chopping at home. Something like butternut squash comes peeled, seeded, and cubed. Those bad boys are tough to cut, and having that work already done saves at least 15 minutes. Cauliflower rice is also a time-saver, as are the bags of broccoli, shredded cabbage, and cleaned and trimmed Brussels sprouts. I know precut can be a little pricier, but it goes a long way. I'll give you more shortcuts in the recipes, but I had to shout-out to my all-star.

One Pot. One Pan. One Love.

The only time you need forty-five dishes clanking around is Thanksgiving, so save your energy for that day. The fewer dishes, the better. And fortunately, there are a lot of delicious cuisines that are possible to make in a pinch. Stews, soups, and even Creamy Mac & Cheese (page 175) all come to life in a big pot, whereas full veggie + protein + carb meals can be made on a single sheet pan and cooked at the same temperature and time.

The one-pan trick also works if you're meal prepping for the week ahead. You can roast various veggies at once on separate sides of the pan, and you're set for the entire week.

Something Out of Nothing

My mom was the queen of opening up the pantry, evaluating the spices on hand, weighing those with the fresh herbs near their end, shaking a box of rice and knowing it was just the right amount to fill each plate, then throwing it all together to make us happy and full.

When Saturday arrives and you're not quite keen on heading to a restaurant, and you've almost used the last bit of food left for the week, I guarantee there is something in there to make a meal. That is, of course, if you have the essentials on hand. It may not seem like it will be the most exciting meal of the week, but like my mom, I, too, have a knack for making something out of nothing, and that includes a fun time. The most important thing is that you're able to call the family to the table to clink forks and chitchat. Pasta, butter, and parmesan night is one to cherish, remember?

It's like when you're out in the woods, camping under the stars, and seeing what you can do with fire and some tinfoil. And typically, even if it's not the most gourmet dish you've ever had in your life, the adventure of it makes up for that. Use this same disposition in your kitchen when you're running low on ingredients and energy. Refer to the flavor combos and mint something new. Dry spices are there to amplify nothing into something. When I'm running low, I refer to my nonrecipe recipes that you can make with what's on hand if you know the basic techniques.

Pesto

One of my all-time favorite "something from nothing" quick fixes is a pesto, the herbaceous green sauce that will accent anything. In Italian, pesto comes from the verb "to pound," because the customary method combines ingredients—a handful of basil, a spoonful of pine nuts, a garlic clove, lemon juice, salt, olive oil, and parmesan—in a mortar and pestle and pounds them into a vibrant paste. It's that type of thing where you know the general idea and wing it. If I'm making a big batch, I'll pull out the food processor or blender. Use pesto on pasta, drizzle over chicken, toss with roasted veggies or rice, or swirl into a soup!

Yield: 2 cups, enough for 1 pound of pasta

- ✳ 2 cups basil or parsley leaves
- ✳ 2 garlic cloves, peeled
- ✳ Juice of 1 medium lemon
- ✳ 2 tablespoons nuts (pine, walnut, cashew, or almond)
- ✳ ⅓ cup grated parmesan (or nutritional yeast)
- ✳ Olive oil or broth, enough to liquefy the mixture

If I'm being real, I just drop in everything and give it a spin. Most of the time I also include ingredients I'm sneaking into everyone's diets:

AVOCADO: This gives it an extra creamy consistency.

LEAFY GREENS: Spinach, kale, and sometimes I'll even use what's left of mixed green salad.

OTHER SOFT HERBS: Mint and chervil

ROOT VEGETABLE LEAVES: Radish leaves work well in this, as do beet greens.

ZUCCHINI: Got a zucchini on the edge? Roughly chop it and blend it in, too. Why not!

Soups

When in doubt or a damsel in dinner distress, soup it out! You can create a soup from basically anything. You just start with the foundational ingredients and layer on from there. Depending on the spices you have on hand, you can really go at it and flavor it however you want. If you have broth in the pantry, a soup will get you through any chilly evening.

BASE SOUP

- Tia's Trinity (1 chopped onion, 1 chopped garlic clove, and 2 tablespoons olive oil)
- 2 cups chopped veggies
- 4 to 6 cups low-sodium broth or stock (veggie or chicken)

FLAVOR ADD-INS

- Roasted chicken (anything that's left from your weekly roast)
- Cooked pasta
- Cooked rice
- No-salt-added canned beans

TWO QUICK FLAVOR IDEAS:

Southwestern

- ½ teaspoon ground cumin
- 1 teaspoon dried oregano
- 1 teaspoon paprika or chili powder
- 1 (14.5-ounce) can diced or crushed tomatoes (optional)

Chicken noodle

- 1 teaspoon dried thyme
- 1 teaspoon dried oregano
- ¼ cup fresh parsley, roughly chopped

Smoothies

My family is a bunch of smoothie enthusiasts. First of all, smoothies are incredibly refreshing, especially during the summer; they pack in loads of vitamins and minerals and are the perfect go-to when I'm pushing produce and slipping in vegetables my kids won't eat when they're whole on a plate. There's no recipe for this, but if you're scraping the bottom of the barrel one night and have only frozen fruits and veggies, heck! Call it a smoothie night! My norm is usually nondairy milk (I prefer almond) with a handful of berries and spinach, a scoop of vanilla protein powder, a drizzle of honey, and either chia seeds, ground flaxseed, or spirulina. If I'm sharing with my kids, I remove the protein powder.

Rice Bowls

A scoop of rice or quinoa topped with veggies (steamed, roasted, leftover!) is both hearty and healthy. Because the possibilities can and will never end here, you can do anything you want quickly. Besides soy sauce, you can make it bright and summery with freshly squeezed lemon juice and olive oil, or top it with your pesto. I love to do a quick trick when the rice is about 15 minutes from being done—I put chopped veggies right on top and steam or heat them up along with the rice.

Chopped Salads

Yes, salads are cooking, and like soups you can make them with whatever your heart desires. I use a mason jar for the dressing ingredients and shake a batch because it lasts for a week or two in the fridge. Having this on hand spares you the additives and unnecessary ingredients typically found in store-bought dressings, like sugar and food coloring (which may be included to give more eye appeal; can you believe it?).

BASE DRESSING
* ½ cup extra-virgin olive oil
* ¼ cup lemon juice
* 2 teaspoons Dijon mustard
* 1 or 2 garlic cloves, minced, pressed, or grated
* Kosher salt and freshly ground black pepper to taste

DRESSING ADD-INS
* Finely chopped fresh herbs (parsley, mint, chervil, marjoram, thyme, anything!)
* Shredded parmesan
* Vinegar (balsamic, white wine, champagne, rice)
* Honey or agave (to balance the acidity)

Chicken Stock

What to do with leftover roast chicken bones and random bits of veggies and herbs? Make stock and freeze it! It's super easy and uses stragglers in the fridge. Once you get the hang of this technique, you'll find yourself subconsciously tossing in whatever you have on hand. Also, it's okay to leave out an ingredient if you don't have it. No need to run to the store for celery! If you just cooked a roast chicken but you're not quite ready for stock prep, wrap up the bones and freeze for later.

* 1 tablespoon olive oil
* Bones of a whole chicken: for example, left over from the Spatchcocked Lemon-Herb Chicken with Roasted Baby Potatoes (page 198) or 3-Ingredient Roasted Chicken (page 207)
* 1 white or yellow onion, quartered (okay to leave the skin on)
* 5 garlic cloves, smashed (okay to leave the skin on)
* 2 carrots, halved
* 2 celery stalks, halved
* Handful of fresh herbs (parsley or thyme are best here) or 2 teaspoons dried herbs (thyme, Italian seasoning, parsley)
* Bay leaf
* 1 teaspoon salt
* 2 teaspoons peppercorns
* 8 cups water

In a large stockpot, heat the olive oil over medium heat. Add the bones, onion, garlic, carrots, celery, herbs, bay leaf, salt, and peppercorns. Sauté for 7 minutes, stirring occasionally. Add the water and bring to a boil over high heat. Reduce to a slow simmer and cook, uncovered, for 1½ hours, stirring occasionally.

Strain the contents of the pot through a fine-mesh sieve and discard the solids. Cool then transfer the stock to airtight plastic containers and refrigerate. Use immediately or freeze for up to 3 months.

Tia's Tips

If you want, skim the fat from the stock before reheating. There won't be too much fat, so this is completely up to you.

It's easy to make this more flavorful by adding a 1-inch piece of fresh ginger, cut in half, or more garlic, onion, carrots, or celery.

TIME CHARTS

Sheet pan roasting: Once you have your sheet pans, you'll never let go—never! For vegetable side dishes, it's often easiest to toss everything in olive oil, salt, and pepper, spread onto a sheet pan, and roast while you prepare the other dinner fixings. For those with the same cooking time, you can combine and cook all at once, as long as they are cut to the same size. Toss halfway through the cooking process.

CHICKEN	SIZE	COOK TIME	OVEN TEMPERATURE	INTERNAL TEMPERATURE
Breast, bone-in, skin-on	6 to 8 ounces	30 to 40 minutes		
Breast, boneless, skinless	4 ounces	20 to 30 minutes		
Drummies	4 ounces	35 to 45 minutes	350°F	165°F
Legs or thighs	4 to 8 ounces	40 to 50 minutes		
Wings	2 to 3 ounces	30 to 40 minutes		

SEAFOOD	SIZE	COOK TIME	OVEN TEMPERATURE	INTERNAL TEMPERATURE
Halibut	5 ounces	12 to 14 minutes		145°F or until flesh is opaque and fish easily flakes with a fork
Sea bass	5 ounces	12 to 14 minutes	400°F	
Snapper	6 ounces	15 to 17 minutes		
Wild salmon	6 ounces	12 to 14 minutes		

PORK	SIZE	COOK TIME	OVEN TEMPERATURE	INTERNAL TEMPERATURE
Chops, bone-in	1½ inch thick	12 to 22 minutes	Broil, 4 to 5 inches from heat	145°F
	¾ inch thick	8 to 12 minutes		
Chops, boneless	1½ inch thick	12 to 22 minutes		
	¾ inch thick	8 to 12 minutes		

ROASTED VEGETABLES	SIZE	COOK TIME	OVEN TEMPERATURE	INTERNAL TEMPERATURE
Asparagus	Whole	10 to 15 minutes, depending on thickness		
Broccoli	1-inch florets	15 to 25 minutes		
Brussels sprouts	Halved	25 to 30 minutes		
Carrots, turnips, and sweet potato (great combo!)	1-inch pieces	30 minutes	400°F	N/A
Cauliflower	1-inch florets	25 to 30 minutes		
Peppers	1-inch pieces	20 minutes		
Summer squash (zucchini and yellow squash)	1-inch rounds	20 to 25 minutes		
Winter squash (butternut, kabocha, pumpkin)	1-inch pieces	25 to 35 minutes		

LITTLE WISDOMS

Julia Child, that firecracker of the kitchen, began her adulthood as an intelligence officer for the CIA. Yes, you read that right. She found her way into cooking during WWII after an assignment to concoct a recipe for an animal-friendly shark repellent. We know what happened next: a lifetime filled with recipe development, entertaining, French cuisine, and educating the masses. She held nothing back and accepted every splash and spill. What made her special was her unapologetic yet affable attitude. She used to say, "No matter what happens in the kitchen, never apologize," which I LOVE. The moment you sit down and say, "Sorry, the Brussels sprouts may be a tad undercooked," people will focus on that announcement and seek out the mistake they probably wouldn't have noticed until you pointed it out. It's okay to be a little coy when you present food to others, but it's also charming to be proud! Not big ego pride, but excited about your job! Even if there *is* a little flaw to conceal.

A few of my favorite tips are ones I stumbled upon along the way, and with each one, I found a new perspective.

CLEANING MUSHROOMS: Dampen a towel and lightly wipe off the dirt. Mushrooms absorb liquid like a sponge, and cleaning them while immersed in water will impact the texture in a not-so-pleasant way.

SEARING MEAT: When searing meat, you're locking in the juices and developing a nice crunch on the outside. Don't touch it before you flip it. Let it do its thing. If you move it around a lot, it won't get that nice sear!

RESTING MEAT: Crucial, crucial, crucial. You worked so hard not to touch the meat so it retains its juices. When taking it out of the oven or off the stove/grill, rest it for 5 to 10 minutes. If you slice into it right away because you're hungry and tempted, the juices that make the meat delicious will be all over your cutting board and not in the meat, resulting in a dried-out or rubbery bite. At Thanksgiving, rest your turkey, too!

GARLIC: Garlic can burn very quickly, and we don't want that happening. Burnt garlic has a yucky taste. When sautéing garlic, keep an eye on it and move it around a lot. If you see it browning too quickly and you're not ready for the next step in the recipe, take it off the heat or out of the pan and set it aside. Another trick is "sweating" it by cooking it on top of another ingredient, like an onion. Got garlic fingers? Rub your digits on a little bit of stainless steel (your kitchen faucet, perhaps) or give them a quick spritz of citrus.

SIFTING DRY INGREDIENTS: When a recipe calls for this step, don't skip it. Sifting breaks up any clumps and makes your batter smooth.

PASTA WATER: When I cook pasta, I always remove about a cup of water from the pot. The starch from the water gives a sauce creaminess and keeps it from drying out. It also thins out a sauce if it's too thick, helping to cover all the pasta noodles. Use ¼ cup at a time to get the consistency right. I don't use pasta water all the time, but I know it's there if I need it.

DRIED HERBS: Before putting them into action, rub the herb between your hands to release more flavor. Then, let it rain into the pot or pan!

BROTH: If a recipe calls for water (say you're cooking rice), you can use broth instead to add more flavor. This is fully up to you when you decide to do it, and there is no rule across the board. If I'm trying to cut back on olive oil in something like pesto, I sub in cold broth. Mashed potatoes? Broth instead of milk. Of course, dinner guests might miss the silky richness that cream provides, but you won't be wobbling from the table afterward.

CREAMY SOUPS: Again, case by case here, but if you want to eliminate heavy creams, blend some of the ingredients with broth. It will thicken the soup and transform from liquid-y to creamy without the guilt.

IMPROV IS FUN: Remember that recipes can be adjusted and if you don't have an ingredient that requires a small quantity, just leave it out.

BACON: To save time and extra dishes, cook an entire package at once. Bacon keeps well in the refrigerator, and you can reheat it quickly in the microwave or oven. Use it for breakfast, in a sandwich, or added to salads or pasta dishes.

ONION: After cutting into an onion, you can store the rest for up to 2 weeks in an airtight container or wrapped very tightly in plastic wrap. Use the leftover onion for cooked recipes, as raw will be too strong.

KID'S KITCHEN

A kitchen is a wondrous place for a child. Children watch their parents navigate shiny utensils as sizzling sounds heighten the soundtrack of the room and enticing fragrances tickle their noses. As you whiz from task to task, whisk in one hand, flour dabbed on your face, and a tune jingling from your mouth, it's a bit of a spectacle. It doesn't take a lot to interest a kid in helping out (unless you ask them to clean, which is a whole different book).

Cooking uses all the senses: smell, touch, hearing, sight, and taste. Involving kids incites learning and development. I know this from my own experience growing up and watching it happen with Cree and Cairo. It's a grand experiment of breaking food down, manipulating its size, texture, shape, and flavor with your own hands. It's whimsical and scientific. When I was a budding cook, I looked forward to trying new foods. I may not have yearned for broccoli, but when mom let me season it, I sampled the darn thing. Eventually, I looked forward to broccoli because I had a hand in the process. Once Cree became old enough, I gave him safe duties like slicing fruits with a butter knife. He now cuts his own bagels and smears on the cream cheese. He's so proud when he does it! For the little ones, bring out colorful bowls and let them stir, stir, stir. The more involved they are, the more they understand. They begin to appreciate food when it goes above and beyond "Sit down and eat this."

Tasks vary from age to age, as do attention spans. Once kids can stand up on their two feet, they can help out. The wee toddlers are still developing motor skills and can take on only basic assignments like pouring and mixing. As I write this book, Cairo says "ladder, ladder" to indicate she wants to help and watch me cut up colorful things. While she stands there, her interest is locked in. Being present in the moment and supporting me gives her a sense of power and bravery that she won't achieve sitting on the couch. She even helps Cory make smoothies by choosing fruits and placing them in the blender. Food-centric

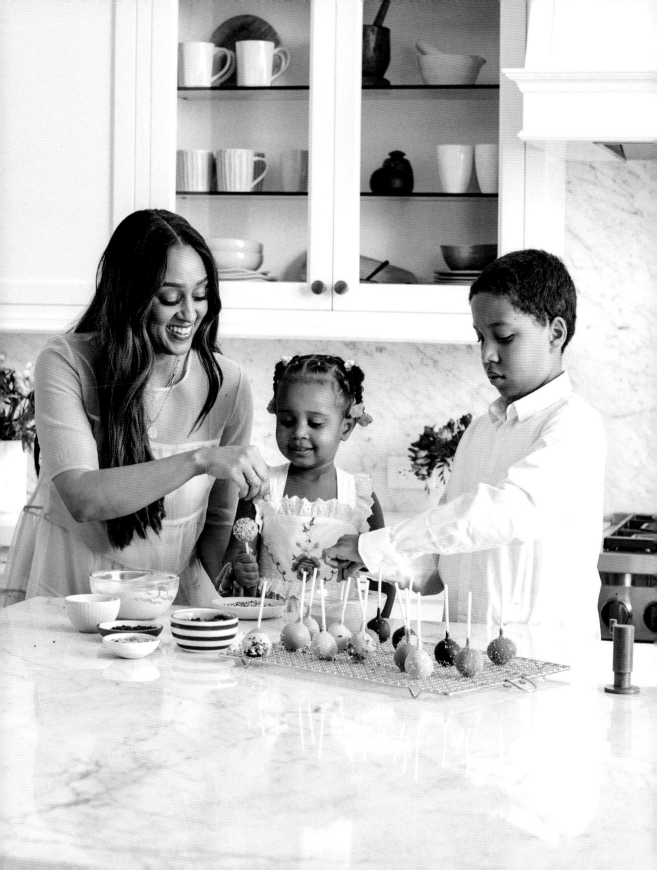

screen time—*MasterChef Junior*, for instance—cultivates further curiosity as children witness their peers tackling the kitchen. My friend's five-year-old daughter is obsessed with that show, and her dream is to meet Chef Gordon Ramsay. The kind, gentle version of him, of course. This just tickles me.

Carve out time when you enlist help from the kids. It will take longer than usual, and happy accidents are bound to happen. If you're under a time constraint, it can add stress and diminish the fun. When Cree graduated to cracking eggs, we accidentally ate a lot of shells, but it was worth seeing the look on his face when he did it by himself, mesmerized by the whites and yolk flowing from the shell to the bowl. Cooking for my siblings back in the day, I felt accomplished, and I can see that confidence forming in Cree, too. Completing a task from start to finish (even if it's just cutting his own bagel) and observing everyone enjoy it is an incredible feat! I imagine that's what Beyoncé feels like when singing to 30,000 people, right?

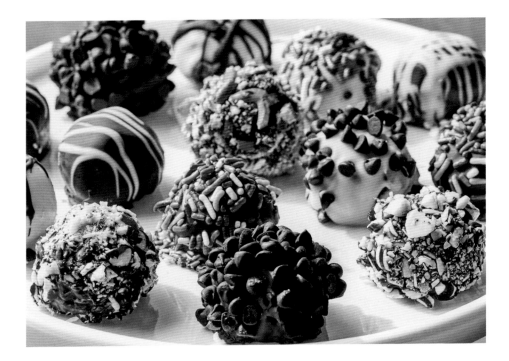

SAFETY FIRST

Teaching the little ones to cook doesn't mean you can pass the buck and forgo kitchen duty. Cooking will help them grow fond of the kitchen, build traditions, and introduce them to new foods. Although the kitchen is an excellent place for learning, it also poses its dangers. I make sure everyone (including me) is fully present and paying attention. For the younger kids, a burst of energy can instantly disengage them and lead to a mishap. Allow them to shake it off somewhere else. For teens, cooking can cycle into chore duties, with periodic pauses for studying and homework.

Make a habit of washing hands before diving in and during the process. Kids may not fully understand what salmonella is, but growing that awareness is critical from the get-go. Gently remind your pint-size chef of the things they can and cannot touch: stove, food/pans straight out of the oven, sharp knives or kitchen shears, and your glass of wine. Let them know the appropriate tasks for kids and why certain things are designated for adults. Present tools slowly as they expand their skills, comfort level, and confidence.

PLAN AHEAD

When I'm meal planning and want Cree's assistance, I call him in so that we can choose a recipe together. I start by asking if there's anything new he wants to experiment with, then we scroll through my cookbooks for an accessible version of it. Let's use Veggie Tamale Pie (page 170) as an example. There isn't too much involvement and I can do the prep work before his chef's cap is on. A recipe like this is great because kids can assemble the ingredients in order without too many tasks. Steer the ship by rinsing the produce and chopping the ingredients. I sometimes measure ahead of time if Cree has a lot of homework (or if his energy level is slumped). This sets us up for a swift preparation without juggling back and forth, searching for tools and ingredients while Cree's attention slips away.

RELAX

Most kids can't keep their rooms clean, let alone the kitchen. Heck, it's hard for me sometimes to maintain tidiness while fixing the nightly meal. Expect this, and don't be surprised if it looks like you two just had a food fight. The journey is more important than keeping the space spick-and-span. While it's imperative to keep a close eye, jumping at every twist and turn may spark a little anxiety. If I'm not comfortable with Cree cutting the veggies, I hold off on handing him the knife until I'm fully ready. Instead, I assign tasks that put us both at ease.

Confidence is something a kid can truly gain here, even if they make a mistake. Kids are destined to mess up in the kitchen. I mess up all the time but keep on keepin' on. When I'm with Cree, I up my pats-on-the-back game and always gently remind him to "dust off and try again." I'm looking at you, Mom!

AGE-FRIENDLY TASKS

AGES 3 TO 4

Ah, the inquisitive age. Curiosity is overflowing from those growing little heads, and enthusiasm for all things is at a constant. "Why this?" "Why that?" It is music to my ears! I love watching babies grow into little humans who ask questions about everything. In the kitchen, this is a pivotal stage of learning and interest.

* Getting tools out
* Washing fruits and vegetables
* Mashing ingredients, like overripe bananas or potatoes
* Layering dishes, such as lasagnas, enchiladas, and baked breakfasts
* Mixing ingredients in bowls, such as pancake, cupcake, or cake batters (they may not have the strength to combine it all, but they'll love trying)
* Sifting (watch their eyes as snow falls from the sifter! Make. It. Rain. Cairo!)

* Rolling dough with guidance
* Shaping cookies with cookie cutters
* Decorating desserts
* Pouring measured ingredients into bowls or a blender

AGES 5 TO 7

Kids are more coordinated and confident in their knowledge at this age, so feel free to up their game according to your and their comfort level. There are a lot of kid-friendly kitchen tools on the market to make tasks safer, like knives with nylon blades. By this age, kids also have more muscle in their arms, which gives them the strength to thoroughly whisk, mix, and mash things. If they're able to read, have them read the steps out loud while you work together!

* Setting the table
* Cracking eggs
* Using a hand mixer
* Scooping cookie dough/batter with the ice cream scooper and placing it on a cookie sheet or in muffin tins
* Rolling meatballs
* Cutting softer fruits and veggies using a kid-friendly knife
* Measuring (great math education here!)
* Cleaning, including loading the dishwasher, sweeping, wiping the table

AGES 8 TO 12

This is when you can start handing over more duties to kids, sit back, and read a book at arm's reach if they need your sous-chef assistance. Lean in to this! If they already showed interest in cooking, they'll probably tell you to leave the kitchen. But I'm keepin' a close eye anyway.

* Peeling veggies
* Using a kid-friendly knife for next-level ingredients, such as bell peppers, apples, and zucchini
* Making sandwiches or tortilla pinwheels
* Washing and putting away dishes
* Unloading groceries
* Toasting and buttering bread (or bagels, like Cree!)

AGES 13 AND UP

At this age, kids will want to take on more tasks and complete meals from start to finish. If they don't necessarily love it, work cooking in as a chore but give them full rein on picking and planning the meal.

* Using sharp knives
* Becoming acquainted with the gadgets: food processors and blender
* Cooking on the stovetop and in the oven

KIDS' TOOLS

I keep tools and utensils in a place accessible for kids so they can help retrieve and put things away.

TODDLER TOWER: Cree loved this when he was little, and Cairo is embracing it with open arms! The tower is a lifted barricade that helps kids reach the counter. The tower is more stable and secure than a chair, and if they reach far for an ingredient, they're locked in and won't fall. From the tower, Cairo helps me cut fruit with a butter knife, makes smoothies with Dad, or watches me scramble eggs.

APRONS: An extra touch that makes them feel like they're putting on a costume, a cooking cloak that gives them confidence and keeps them clean. Well, cleaner than without it. There are so many fun aprons online for every size and age.

CHEF'S HAT: They may not wear it past the age of five, but I know when Cairo crowns herself with the hat, she perks up and knows her job!

COLORFUL SPOONS AND BOWLS: Incorporating color brings that added excitement kids love and makes it easier when dictating instructions. It's clearer to say "get the green bowl" rather than "get the medium-size bowl." Choose appealing colors and tailor the tools to heighten their interest. If your kid likes football, and you stumble upon bowls with footballs on them . . . touchdown!

KID-SIZE TOOLS: I found tasks are more manageable for the small humans if the tools fit their size; this can mean finding a kid's whisk, spatula, and/or spoons. They're easier for those bitsy hands to grip and control.

TRYING NEW FOODS

People always comment on how great my kids eat, that they're adventurous and enjoy foods their kids usually throw on the floor. It's actually one of my favorite compliments I receive! I don't stray from introducing exotic flavors to my kids, and if they don't like them right off the bat, I shrug my shoulders and try again some other time. Because of this, they have advanced palates and a willingness to explore.

One time, Cree sat on the counter and helped me blend up a veggie-centric spicy green smoothie. I'm talking fresh ginger, lemon, kale, avocado, cucumber, and banana. As he watched the ingredients swirl from solid to a luscious smoothie, his eyes widened with wonder. When I poured it into my glass, he asked to try some. I chuckled internally because I had a feeling he would hate it, but I didn't want to deny him! He took a big gulp and cringed as one of those forced smiles reached from cheek to cheek. "Oh" is all he said before jumping to the floor and running to the other room. Do I think he'll try my salad in a cup again anytime soon? Probably not, but glad he gave it a go! When I was a kid, I hated onions. They grossed me out. I meticulously dug through my food to pick out any onion remnants as if I was searching for gold. Gross, pungent gold. Not anymore, though! If I don't have onions in the house, it's because I'm sick and didn't go to the store that week or I'm out of town. And I'm proud to say that my kids eat them without complaint because I'm sly and sauté them until they're melt-in-your-mouth soft.

When I'm introducing new foods, I either do it in very small portions to not overwhelm the child or I get crafty. It's the one time I tell my kids to leave the room so I can covertly accomplish my mission. When I first started giving Cairo broccoli, she swatted the florets off her highchair like a ninja, and I have to say it was quite impressive how far they flew. So, I knew broccoli would be a delicate dance with her. What I do is combine the new food with a food she already loves. In this case, I blend broccoli into mashed potatoes (steamed cauliflower works like a charm for this, too!) and together we marvel at the fact that I made green mashed potatoes! She is none the wiser, but she is healthier. Eventually, her taste buds familiarized themselves with broccoli's flavor, and now she's quite fond of it. In fact, she stands on her ladder and helps me cut it and nibbles away in the process.

Pizza is another way to slip in the nutrients. If Cree could eat pizza every day for breakfast, lunch, and dinner, he would, and to be candid, I would, too. Luckily, I have recipes in this book that allow that, but to my point, I recently made homemade pizza and topped it with fennel, onion, and sausage. The second Cree caught wind of the pizza scent, he ran down to the kitchen for a slice. When I handed it to him, he pointed to the strange substance on top and questioned it. I began thoroughly explaining the derivation of fennel. He immediately nodded and devoured the slice as if it were his last. And there he was, enjoying fennel.

Here are some other devious ways to blend in the veggies:

MEATBALLS: Grate veggies into the mixture. Zucchini is great because it keeps the meatballs moist.

RICE: Mix in peeled and shredded zucchini, finely chopped cauliflower, or even kale/spinach "confetti" (make sure to call it confetti).

PASTA: Try spiralized zucchini noodles or orange butternut squash noodles (you can buy this premade) and celebrate the bright colors that these fun pastas have to offer.

FRUIT SMOOTHIES: Start with a fruit base and give them the Hulk treatment with kale, spinach, or avocado.

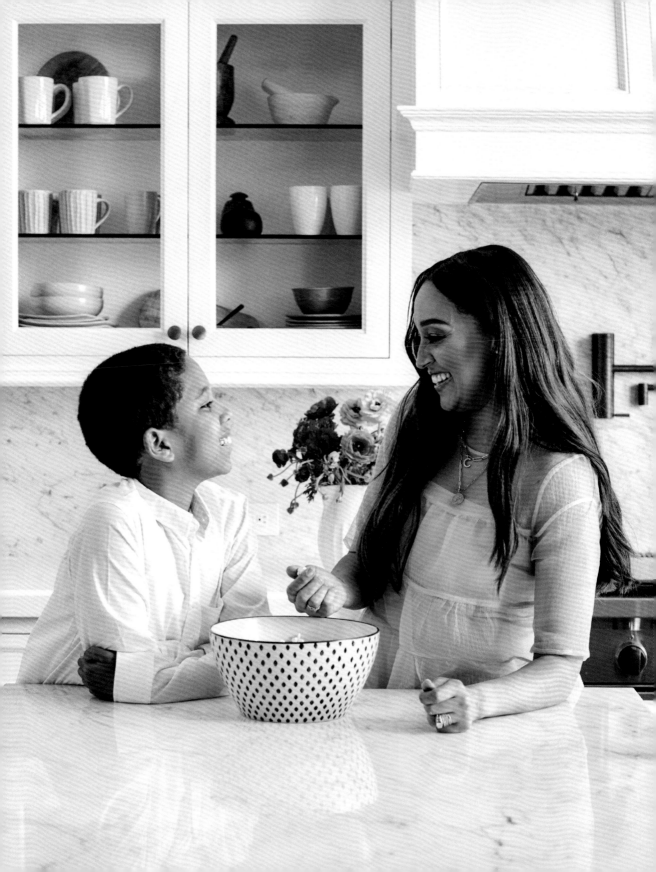

NOURISHED KITCHEN

nourish ⚹ verb; used with object / nour·ish /
to sustain with food or nutriment; supply with what is necessary for life, health, and growth.
to cherish, foster, keep alive. to strengthen, build up, or promote

It's almost time to eat!

My favorite nights are when I incorporate the family into the process. When I didn't have kids, Cory and I made one night a week a stay-at-home date night and tackled a new recipe together. If you're single? Put on heels and your cutest apron and treat yourself!

My ritual of gathering the family around the table strengthens our bond. Cooking is rooted in tradition. Food is an inherent tool for handing down traditions, even if they are solely for yourself. Every year, the day after Thanksgiving, I eat apple pie à la mode for breakfast. Every year for decades. This is my personal ritual. Some families may play a game of tag football on Christmas Day, a tradition passed down through generations. And the story keeps being told.

Honoring this lineage *is* family. The most habitual act is eating together. Not only does it feed the soul, but it also nourishes the body. When both are full and balanced, I know that I am in a good place, especially when my family unit is strong. Because when they are, I am. When I feel weak, they use their energy to lift me up and balance me. Eating together is being present with one another and checking in with your family. While sharing my mom's collard greens, we share our story: "Mom, I had a great day, but I'm struggling with math." Or, "Hubby, I'm stressed at work. More wine, please." Without these moments, the connection wouldn't be balanced. When cooking these recipes, remember this and when you bring the food to the table, bring a story, too.

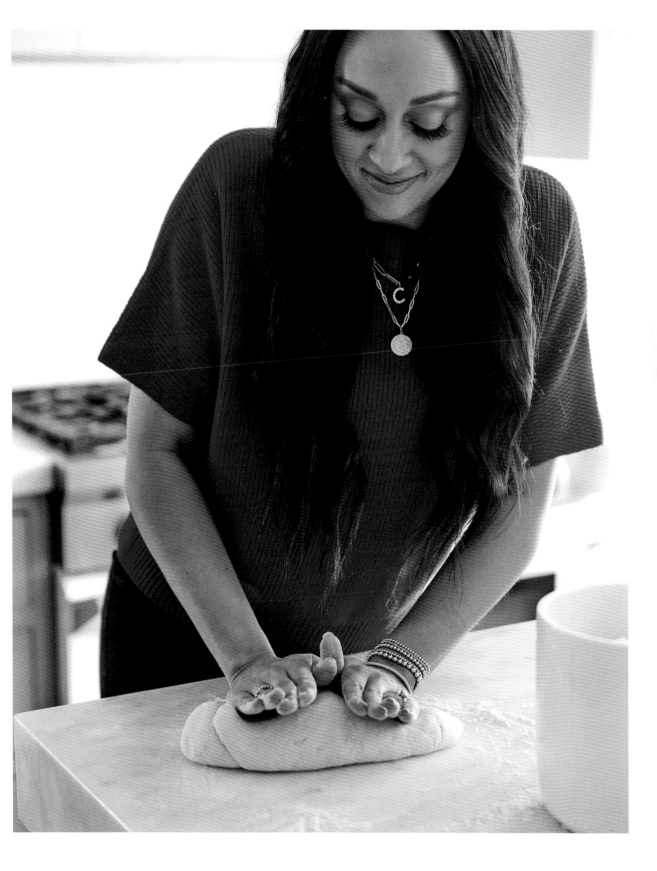

SETTING THE TABLE

Much like my own upbringing, our table is center stage. Before gathering, I like to fill it with the props needed to eat. Or better yet, I like to have Cree handle it for us. We don't overdo it unless it's a holiday, then I let loose, and no one can stop me! For our everyday evenings, however, I keep it simple. Cree places utensils in a pitcher and lays down the plates, napkins, and cups. It doesn't look magazine-perfect, but creating the unity and group effort makes it special. Setting the table tags it as a "formal" event.

No, not black-tie formal, but an official ringing of the bell letting everyone know it's time to gather.

For holidays, it's a whole other story. I love the wow factor of a tablescape, bringing colors from the season onto the table, writing little name cards to assign seats, bundling flowers in the spring and summer and pine cones, twigs, and colored leaves during the fall. It's making the table the star of the show, which makes guests feel special, too.

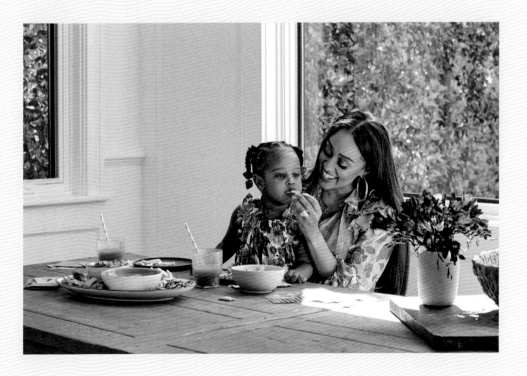

PRESENTATION

No need to pull out those garnish tweezers to plate an extraordinary piece of art, just give the plate some love and attention. We eat with our eyes first. If something appears as a heap of mud on a plate, no one is going to say, "Oh, that looks delicious. Give it to me immediately!" They'll probably decline and fake a headache. Don't get wound up about the presentation but make it *presentable*. I'm always saying, "Make it prrreetttty!" which basically means make it look appetizing and enticing. A thoughtful presentation shows my diners that they're in for a real treat.

In elementary school, I would stare at the clock neurotically while the minute hand snail-crawled its way to lunchtime. When that bell rang, I'd be the first one out the door, eager to eat my lunch. I try to reimagine that excitement for my kids at home, too; every meal is a joyous occasion they look forward to. Kids definitely use their eyes to determine whether or not they want to dig in. The more color, the more exciting it can be. I sometimes cut things into little shapes, making food fun and giving the wee one a reason to grab hold and enjoy. I also try not to overcrowd the plate because it may overwhelm them if they think there's more than they can consume. Make it light!

Drumroll pleeaasssseee! Now it's time to eat. Sit down with your loved ones and do your first *Quick Fix* menu plan together. Dog-ear pages, scribble notes, and remember that this book absorbs all spills that come its way. I truly hope you enjoy cooking the recipes in this book as much as I did writing them for you. Bon appétit!

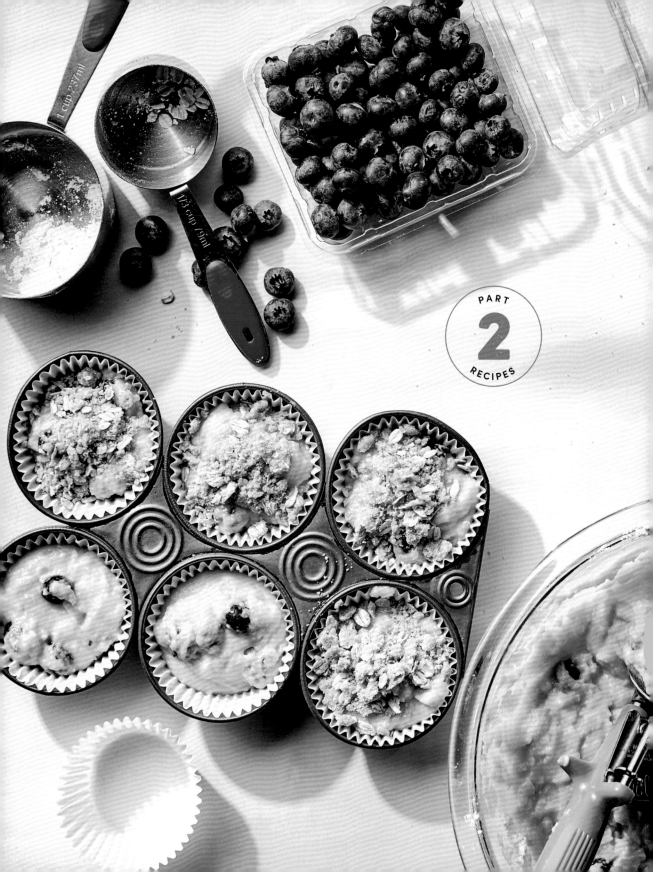

Breakfast

Sheet PanCakes

SERVES 8
PREP TIME: 15 minutes
TOTAL TIME: 25 minutes

2 cups dairy milk or unsweetened nut milk

2 teaspoons apple cider vinegar or distilled white vinegar

½ cup (1 stick) unsalted butter, melted

2 cups all-purpose flour

⅔ cup cornstarch

1 tablespoon baking powder

1 teaspoon baking soda

1 teaspoon ground cinnamon (optional)

½ teaspoon kosher salt

2 large eggs, whisked

2 teaspoons pure vanilla extract

OPTIONAL TOPPINGS

Sliced bananas

Blueberries, fresh or frozen

Sliced strawberries

Raspberries

Chocolate chips

Toasted coconut flakes

Let me introduce my best friend, the sheet pan (or rimmed baking sheet or sheet tray, whatever you want to call it), with which you will become more acquainted throughout this book. I bet you never imagined making pancakes this way, but with a sheet pan, the possibilities are endless. This recipe is a perfect example of quick fixing: It's fun, it easily caters to everyone's preferences in one fell swoop, lets kids go wild, and offers up a group activity for everyone!

In a 2-cup measuring cup, combine the milk and vinegar. Whisk and set aside.

Preheat the oven to 425°F. Generously brush an 11 × 17-inch sheet pan with 4 tablespoons of the melted butter.

In a large bowl, sift the flour, cornstarch, baking powder, baking soda, cinnamon (if using), and salt. Make a well in the center of the dry ingredients and add the eggs, vanilla, remaining 4 tablespoons melted butter, and milk/vinegar mixture. Mix until just until combined. Do not overmix.

RECIPE + INGREDIENTS CONTINUE

Tia's Tips

So, what's the deal with overmixing? It overactivates whatever batter you are making. In this case, it will leave pancakes heavy, so mix only until the ingredients are combined. If you think you've overmixed, let the batter rest for 10 minutes before pouring it on the pan.

This relaxes the gluten in the flour, bringing back the light fluffiness we all love about pancakes.

Sifting dry ingredients helps break up any clumps and gives your batter a smoother texture.

FOR SERVING

Maple syrup

Cut-up fresh fruit

Pour the batter into the prepared sheet pan and spread evenly, making one big rectangular pancake. Arrange any desired toppings on the batter, mix them up, separate them, have the kids go to town.

Bake until golden brown and a toothpick in the center comes out clean, 8 to 10 minutes, rotating the pan halfway through. Remove from the oven and let sit for a few minutes. Cut into squares. Serve with maple syrup and more fresh fruit on the side.

If there are leftover pancakes in the pan, let cool completely. Place in an airtight container and freeze for up to 3 months. To serve, remove from the freezer and reheat in the oven or microwave before serving.

Ham & Cheese Puffs

SERVES 6
PREP TIME: 10 minutes
TOTAL TIME: 25 minutes

Nonstick cooking spray

6 slices sandwich bread

3 slices deli ham, halved

6 tablespoons shredded cheddar cheese

4 large eggs

½ teaspoon kosher salt

¼ teaspoon freshly ground black pepper

Fresh parsley, for garnish (optional)

Tia's Tips

These cheese puffs freeze well after cooking! Just wrap individually and pop in the freezer; they'll be good for up to 3 months. Heat in a 375°F oven straight from the freezer and take on the go.

Double this recipe to make a full muffin tin.

Use this recipe as a base to satisfy your heart's desires. Once you have the basics down, throw in your favorite fillings, veggies, or proteins to make it your own.

Preheat the oven to 375°F. Spritz 6 cups of a standard muffin tin or 6 ramekins with cooking spray.

Place the bread on a cutting surface. On one side of the bread, midway from the corners, cut a slit into the center of each slice. Place the slices over the wells in the muffin tins (or the ramekins) and use the slit to curve the bread over so it fits into each cup. Push down to keep in place. Don't worry if your bread breaks, just fill it in to form a cup in the muffin tin.

Line each bread cup with a half-slice of ham. Add 1 tablespoon cheddar. Set aside.

In a small bowl, whisk the eggs, salt, and pepper. Divide the eggs among the 6 muffin cups. If there is any egg left over, let the bread sit for a minute or two so the bread can soak up some of the egg mixture, then you can add the remaining egg.

Transfer to the oven and bake until the center is just set, 15 to 18 minutes. Remove from the oven and let rest for 2 minutes. Run a knife around the edges of the muffin cups or ramekins. Top with fresh parsley for garnish, if using. Remove to a plate and serve.

Use liners in the muffin tins for easier cleanup.

This recipe can be made gluten-free easily! Just check to see if the oats are marked "gluten-free."

Baked Oatmeal Muffins

MAKES 11 OR 12 MUFFINS
PREP TIME: 15 minutes
TOTAL TIME: 45 minutes

Nonstick cooking spray (optional)

2 cups old-fashioned rolled oats

1 teaspoon baking powder

½ teaspoon ground cinnamon

½ teaspoon kosher salt

2 large eggs, whisked

½ cup dairy milk or
    unsweetened nut milk

¼ cup maple syrup or honey

2 tablespoons unsalted butter
    or coconut oil, melted

2 tablespoons creamy nut butter,
    such as peanut, almond,
    or cashew

1 teaspoon pure vanilla extract

Favorite jam or jelly

OPTIONAL TOPPINGS

Berries

Banana

Applesauce

Chopped nuts

Chocolate chips

This is one of those recipes that keeps my belly full until lunch or gets me through an afternoon slump. It has the perfect combination of carbs, good fats, and protein to keep me movin' and groovin'! And like so many of the other recipes in this book, you can please everyone in the household by individualizing the toppings for each muffin!

Preheat the oven to 375°F. Line a muffin tin with liners or spritz a 9 × 9-inch baking dish with cooking spray.

In a large bowl, mix the oats, baking powder, cinnamon, and salt until fully combined.

In another bowl, whisk the eggs, milk, maple syrup, melted butter, nut butter, and vanilla. Add to the oatmeal mixture and stir until fully combined. Using a large ice cream scoop, fill two-thirds of each liner with the oat mixture, making sure it doesn't overflow as these will slightly rise when baking. Top with a heaping teaspoon of jam or jelly (and/or any of the optional toppings: fruit, nuts, chocolate, or any combination you like). (Alternatively, if using a 9 x 9-inch baking dish, pour the batter into the pan. Evenly dollop 1 teaspoon of jam or jelly on top of the batter in 3 rows of 4.)

Bake until the center is set and a toothpick inserted into a muffin comes out clean, 20 to 25 minutes. Remove from the oven. Let sit for 2 minutes before serving. Alternatively, if using a baking dish, bake for an extra 5 to 10 minutes and evenly cut into squares with the jam being in the center. Serve warm.

Store in an airtight container in the refrigerator.

Baked French Toast

SERVES 6 TO 8

PREP TIME: 15 minutes

TOTAL TIME: 8 hours 55 minutes

1 tablespoon unsalted butter

10 cups 1-inch pieces day-old
    bread (cut or torn)

8 large eggs

3 cups whole milk (or your
    favorite nondairy alternative)

2 tablespoons honey

1 teaspoon pure vanilla extract

1 teaspoon ground cinnamon

½ teaspoon kosher salt

1 pound strawberries,
    hulled and sliced

1½ cups blueberries

Maple syrup or honey, for serving

Mornings are coziest when my family shovels this onto their plates. The house smells like a bakery and everyone is super excited to dig in. This recipe is incredibly versatile and well balanced: You get protein from the eggs, and the fruity goodness is just sweet enough that processed sugar is unnecessary. I also love it because it holds for several days with leftovers made easy!

Grease a 9 × 13-inch baking dish with the butter. Add the bread cubes to the dish.

In a large bowl or blender, mix the eggs, milk, honey, vanilla, cinnamon, and salt until well combined. Pour over the bread. Gently mix until the bread is coated completely with the egg mixture. Top with the strawberries and blueberries. Cover with foil and refrigerate overnight.

Preheat the oven to 375°F.

Remove from the refrigerator and bake for 35 to 40 minutes. Remove the foil and continue cooking until the top is golden brown, 5 to 7 minutes. Remove from the oven and serve with maple syrup or honey.

Tia's Tips

Any bread will work in this casserole: leftover hamburger buns, sliced bread ends, gluten-free variations, etc. It can be torn unevenly, so invite the kids in on it!

Use whatever fruit is in season or go for frozen. If you want bananas, add right before baking rather than the night before. This will help avoid browning and an overripened flavor.

Variation

Make this savory by omitting the honey, vanilla, and cinnamon and substituting cooked veggies or sausage and shredded cheese for the fruit.

Soft Scrambled Eggs
with Crispy Bacon

SERVES 2

PREP TIME: 5 minutes

TOTAL TIME: 12 minutes

4 large eggs

1 tablespoon unsalted butter

½ teaspoon kosher salt

¼ teaspoon freshly ground
   black pepper

Oven-Baked Bacon
   (recipe follows)

Toast

Oh, how I love soft scrambled eggs! The creamy, velvety texture is incredibly satisfying and reminds me of France, swirling a torn-off piece of baguette around my plate to sop up the eggs. They are so dang good, you can eat them alone, on toast, in a sandwich or breakfast taco, or with small snips of chives as you daydream of Paris. If you prefer not to use butter when cooking eggs, give the pan a good spritz of cooking spray.

In a medium bowl, whisk the eggs until creamy and slightly frothy along the edges.

In a 10-inch nonstick skillet, melt the butter over medium-low heat. Once the butter has melted, add the whisked eggs. Watch for the edges to just barely start to set. Using a heat-resistant silicone spatula, slowly stir the eggs, from the outside edge of the eggs to the middle, forming large soft curds as the eggs cook. Don't flip over the curds. Repeat the same stir around the outside of the eggs, pausing in between to allow the eggs to cook slightly. This process should take 2 to 3 minutes or less. Do not overcook—look for creamy and shiny eggs.

Transfer to plates and season with salt and pepper. Serve with a few slices of bacon and toast.

RECIPE CONTINUES

OVEN-BAKED BACON

SERVES 4 OR 5

1 pound bacon

Preheat the oven to 400°F.

Line two sheet pans with parchment paper. Arrange the bacon strips on the paper, making sure they do not overlap. You can lay the strips close to one another because they will shrink while cooking. Roast for 7 to 8 minutes and flip each piece. Return to the oven and cook until both sides are crispy, another 5 to 6 minutes. Remove from the oven and let cool. Store any extra bacon in an airtight container in the refrigerator and enjoy for the rest of the week! Just microwave for 30 seconds and serve.

Tia's Tips

For eggs, I strongly suggest using a nonstick skillet, otherwise the eggs will easily crust along the edges and make the pan a pain to clean. Also, the silicone spatula is like a magic wand for eggs, delicately running along the sides of the pan in a way a normal spatula cannot.

Go low and slow. The eggs will transform from perfect to overcooked in a matter of seconds, so keep the flame on low. Also, more stirring results in smaller curds and can dry out the eggs. Be patient, it's worth it.

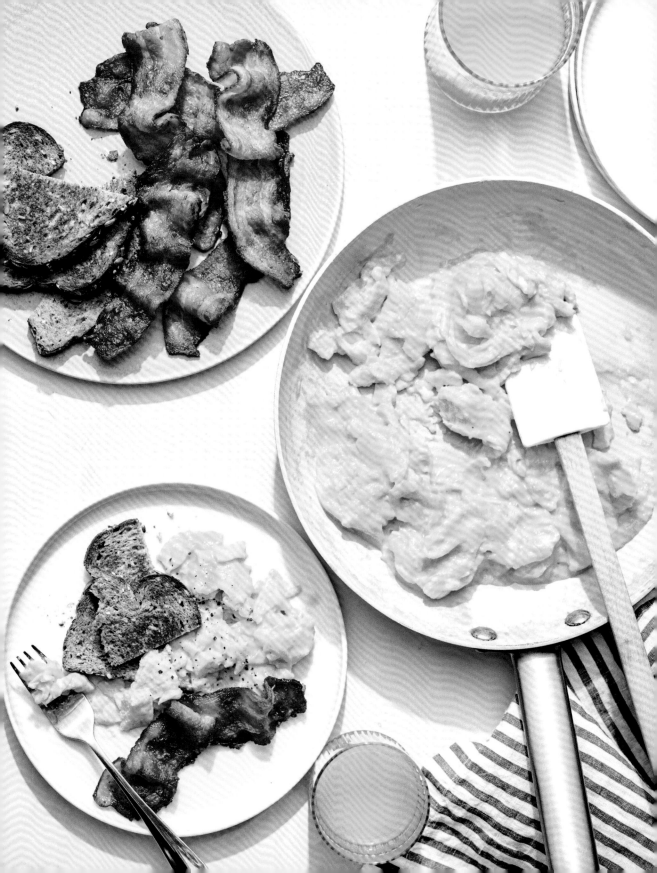

Tia's Tip

Hash browns can be thawed in the fridge overnight or placed in a bowl and microwaved on high for 3 to 4 minutes, stirring twice in between.

Crispy Parmesan Hash Browns

SERVES 4

PREP TIME: 10 minutes

TOTAL TIME: 25 minutes

2 tablespoons extra-virgin olive oil

1 large onion, grated

1 green bell pepper, grated

1 large zucchini, grated (optional)

1 (28-ounce) package frozen shredded hash brown potatoes, thawed

1 teaspoon kosher salt, plus more to taste

½ teaspoon freshly ground black pepper, plus more to taste

4 large eggs

¼ cup grated parmesan or shredded cheddar cheese

Parsley, for garnish (optional)

Take out that box grater and roll up your sleeves, because this recipe has you grating all sorts of things! Box-grating veggies, especially for a dish like this, helps create the same shape and size as the potatoes. Even with my sharp knife and ninja chopping skills, I don't have time to cut everything into little slivers. This, like a lot of my recipes, is easily adapted, so get imaginative and use whatever veggies you like!

Preheat the oven to 400°F.

In a large ovenproof skillet, heat the oil over medium heat. When hot, add the onion, bell pepper, and zucchini (if using). Sauté until soft, about 5 minutes.

Add the hash browns, salt, and pepper and stir. Push the hash browns down into the skillet with the back of a spatula and let sit for 1 minute, then stir. Repeat this process for 8 to 10 minutes. By letting the hash browns sit for 1 minute at a time, you are allowing them to get crispy and golden brown.

Spread the hash browns evenly in the pan. Using the back of a spoon, make 4 wells in the hash browns and crack an egg into each of the wells. Transfer the skillet to the oven and cook until the eggs are set, about 5 minutes. Sprinkle with the cheese and top with parsley (if using). Season with more salt and pepper. Serve immediately.

Blueberry Lemon Muffins

MAKES 18 OR 19 MUFFINS
PREP TIME: 15 minutes
TOTAL TIME: 30 minutes

Nonstick cooking spray

1½ cups all-purpose flour

½ cup granulated sugar

2 teaspoons baking powder

1 teaspoon kosher salt

3 large eggs, at room
temperature

Grated zest and juice of 1 lemon

1½ cups part-skim ricotta cheese

½ cup honey

½ cup (1 stick) unsalted butter,
melted

1 cup frozen or fresh blueberries

TOPPING

½ cup all-purpose flour

½ cup old-fashioned rolled oats

½ cup packed light brown sugar

¼ teaspoon kosher salt

4 tablespoons (½ stick) cold
unsalted butter, cut into
small cubes

These muffins are so moist and flavorful. You can substitute any fruit, but blueberries are great because of their size! Just cut the other fruit into pea-size shapes.

Preheat the oven to 350°F. Line 18 or 19 cups of two muffin tins with paper liners. Lightly spritz the liners with cooking spray.

In a large bowl, whisk together the flour, granulated sugar, baking powder, and salt until combined. In another bowl, whisk the eggs, lemon zest, lemon juice, ricotta, honey, and melted butter until fully mixed. Stir the wet ingredients into the dry ingredients until combined. Don't overmix. Gently fold in the blueberries.

Scoop the batter into the prepared muffin cups, filling them three-quarters of the way up. Set aside.

MAKE THE TOPPING: In a small bowl, whisk together the flour, oats, brown sugar, and salt. With a fork, mash the cold butter cubes into the dry ingredients. It should be fully combined and crumbly. Top each muffin with 1 tablespoon of the topping.

Transfer to the oven and bake until a toothpick inserted into a muffin comes out clean and the tops are golden brown, 15 to 20 minutes. Remove from the oven and place the tins on a wire rack. Allow to cool completely before serving. Store at room temperature for 3 to 5 days in an airtight container.

Tia's Tips

I like to combine sugar and honey. It doesn't make the muffins too sweet, but I feel a bit better about giving it to the kids.

This topping is great for Dutch apple pie, French toast casserole, sweet quick breads (see page 246), or any type of muffins.

The ricotta in this gives it such a dense, rich, and moist texture. In a pinch, sub with 1 cup buttermilk (or the buttermilk swap; see page 73).

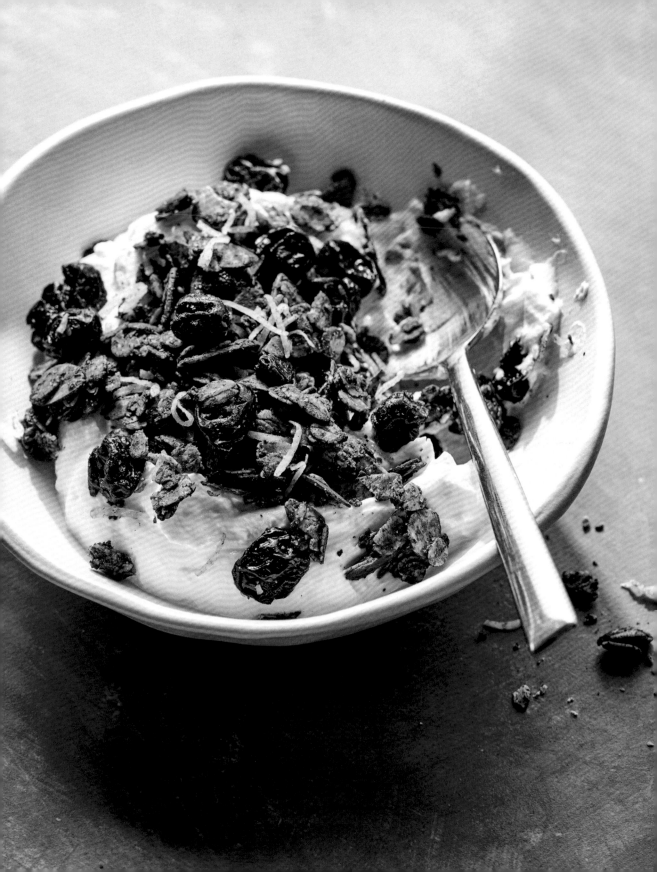

Chocolate Cherry Granola

SERVES 8
PREP TIME: 10 minutes
TOTAL TIME: 35 minutes

4 cups old-fashioned rolled oats

1 cup sliced almonds

¼ cup unsweetened cacao powder

1 teaspoon ground cinnamon

1 teaspoon kosher salt

½ cup coconut oil or unsalted butter (1 stick), melted

½ cup honey

¼ cup nut butter, such as peanut, cashew, almond, or sunflower

1 teaspoon pure vanilla extract

½ cup dried cherries

½ cup shredded coconut, unsweetened or sweetened

Tia's Tips

The granola will crisp up as it cools, so don't feel discouraged when you pull it out of the oven and the texture isn't quite like granola yet; it will get there.

Serve over yogurt, add on top of your favorite smoothie bowl, eat it like cereal with your favorite milk, nibble as a midday snack, or sprinkle on top of ice cream.

Granola is one of my all-time favorite breakfasts, snacks, and grazing foods. Did I say I also love it for dessert? Because I do. However, traditional granola often contains so much sugar, it makes me feel groggy. Granola should be nourishing, so I've created the best of both worlds. If you want sweet, you've got it in the honey and dried fruit. If you want filling, the nut butter adds protein and great flavor. The granola also forms scrumptious clusters that I personally cannot resist! Use any type of nuts, seeds, and dried fruit you like. And if you're feeling extra spirited, add chocolate chips after it has cooled.

Preheat the oven to 350°F. Line a sheet pan with parchment paper.

In a large bowl, stir together the oats, almonds, cacao powder, cinnamon, and salt.

In another bowl, whisk together the oil, honey, nut butter, and vanilla until fully combined. Pour over the oat mixture and mix well, until every oat and nut is coated. Pour the granola onto the lined sheet pan and spread into an even layer.

Bake until lightly golden, 22 to 24 minutes, stirring halfway through and pressing the granola down onto the pan. Remove from the oven and let the granola cool completely. Add the cherries and shredded coconut, tossing and breaking up into clumps.

Store the granola in an airtight container at room temperature for 1 to 2 weeks, or in a sealed freezer bag in the freezer for up to 3 months.

Breakfast Pizza, Two Ways

EACH PIZZA SERVES 8
PREP TIME: 10 minutes
TOTAL TIME: 40 minutes

Extra-virgin olive oil

1 pound store-bought
  pizza dough, at room
  temperature
  (or homemade dough,
  see page 238)

All-purpose flour, for rolling the
  dough

SAVORY PIZZA TOPPINGS

6 large eggs, soft scrambled
  (see Soft Scrambled Eggs with
  Crispy Bacon, page 135)

2 cups frozen potato tots, thawed

1 cup shredded cheddar cheese

8 slices Oven-Baked Bacon
  (page 136), chopped

Kosher salt and freshly ground
  black pepper

Cree's wish has come true: pizza in the evening, then again in the morning! Also, did you ever cook breakfast for dinner growing up? My family loved it so much; it felt incredibly special and crazy. Here's dinner for breakfast, and no, it's not cold leftover pizza.

FOR BOTH PIZZAS: Preheat the oven to 450°F. Drizzle a pizza pan or sheet pan generously with extra-virgin olive oil.

Place the pizza dough on a lightly floured surface. Using clean fingertips, push down into the dough, creating dimples. Flip over and lightly flour again. Pick up the dough and gently stretch it with clean hands. Once you have it to the desired size, place on the prepared pan.

FOR THE SAVORY PIZZA: Transfer the pizza pan to the oven and bake until the edges and crust are golden brown, 15 to 20 minutes.

While the dough is parbaking, make the scrambled eggs, using 1½ tablespoons of butter, and set aside.

Remove the parbaked crust from the oven. Top with the potato tots. With a fork, smash the tots and spread evenly across the top of the crust. Top with the soft scrambled eggs, cheddar, and bacon. Return to the oven until the cheese has melted and the bacon is sizzling, about 5 minutes.

RECIPE + INGREDIENTS CONTINUE

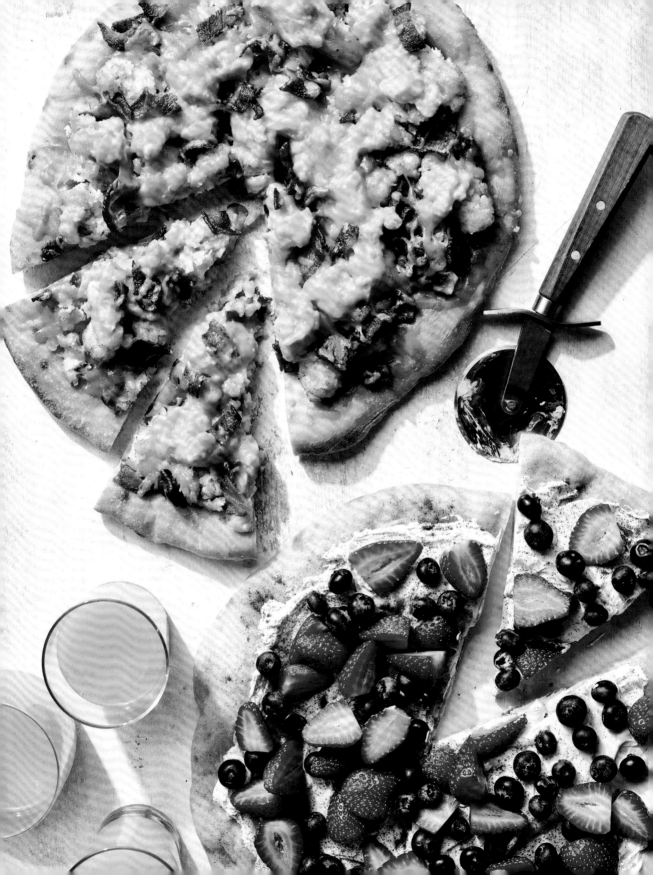

SWEET PIZZA TOPPINGS

½ cup whipped cream cheese

½ teaspoon ground cinnamon

3 to 3½ cups assorted berries, rinsed and dried

1 to 2 tablespoons honey

Pinch of kosher salt

Remove the pizza from the oven to a cutting board. Season with salt and pepper. Slice and serve. This pizza stores well in an airtight container in the refrigerator for 5 to 6 days.

FOR THE SWEET PIZZA: Transfer the pizza pan to the oven and bake until the edges are lightly golden brown, 12 to 15 minutes.

Remove the parbaked crust and spread with whipped cream cheese. The heat of the dough makes spreading the cream cheese easier. Sprinkle with the cinnamon and top with the berries. Drizzle with the honey and salt. Return to the oven and bake for another 8 to 10 minutes; the berries should be soft and shiny.

Remove from the oven and place on a cutting board. Slice and serve. Store any leftovers in an airtight container in the refrigerator for 3 to 4 days.

Tia's Tips

These recipes make great leftovers (lunch, snack, and dinner for Cree!). Place on a baking sheet and heat in the oven at 350°F until warm. Or, if you can't wait, warm in the microwave for 1 minute.

To make the sweet pizza easier for the kiddos, slightly smash the fruit before putting in the oven. This actually creates that gooey jammy texture that I love!

If using strawberries as a topping for the sweet pizza, hull and slice them first.

Frittata in a Cup

SERVES 1

PREP TIME: 5 minutes

TOTAL TIME: 6 minutes 30 seconds

2 large eggs

1 tablespoon milk

Pinch of kosher salt

Freshly ground black pepper

Variations (ingredients follow)

Toast or fruit, for serving

By eating protein with good fats and carbohydrates for breakfast, I'm actually set until lunch. This one-cup meal is perfect for that and is SO EASY to re-create with whatever you're in the mood for. Mexican frittata? *Sí!* Italian frittata? *Perchè no?* Use leftover breads, tortillas, potatoes, or rice. Even pasta will work. I'm giving you the base ingredients and techniques, followed by swaps to inspire you to think outside the cup.

In a large microwave-safe mug, whisk the eggs, milk, salt, and pepper to taste. Stir in the ingredients from your chosen variation. Microwave on high for 1 minute 25 seconds. Remove the mug. If the egg mixture seems wet, return to the microwave for another 10 seconds, until light and fluffy. Let sit for a few minutes before serving. Serve with toast or fruit.

RECIPE CONTINUES

Variations

BACON, POTATO & CHEESE FRITTATA

2 slices bacon, cooked and chopped

2 smashed potato tots

1 tablespoon shredded cheddar cheese

VEGGIE DELIGHT FRITTATA

5 baby spinach leaves, chopped

3 baby tomatoes, chopped

1 tablespoon crumbled goat cheese or shredded
   mozzarella cheese

HAM & CHEESE FRITTATA

2 slices deli ham, slivered

1 slice toast, torn into small pieces

1 tablespoon shredded sharp cheddar cheese

ITALIAN FRITTATA

2 tablespoons tomato sauce

1 tablespoon shredded mozzarella cheese

Top with chopped fresh basil

MEXICAN FRITTATA

2 tablespoons rinsed canned black beans

1 tablespoon salsa

1 tablespoon shredded cheese

½ corn tortilla, torn into small pieces

Milk & Cereal Bars "On the Go"

MAKES 16 BARS

PREP TIME: 10 minutes

TOTAL TIME: 4 to 8 hours

3 cups honey-sweetened Greek yogurt or sweetened nondairy yogurt

2 to 2½ cups store-bought cereal or granola

Tia's Tips

You can also use unsweetened plain yogurt here and mix in 1 to 2 tablespoons honey.

Add nuts or seeds to the cereal mixture for more protein and a crunchy texture.

Honestly, this could pass for dessert, but it's breakfast! It's basically a bowl of cereal on the go. You can wrap each bar with parchment paper and snag when you're running late or dealing with a case of the Mondays.

Line a 9 × 9-inch baking dish with parchment paper in both directions, so it overhangs by 2 inches on all four sides. This will help to easily remove the bars after freezing.

Evenly spread the yogurt into the bottom of the dish. Sprinkle the cereal onto the yogurt. Using a clean hand or the back of the measuring cup, gently press the cereal into the yogurt so it will freeze together.

Cover with plastic wrap and place in the freezer until frozen solid, 4 to 8 hours. Remove the bars from the dish by lifting up the sides of the parchment paper and place on a cutting board. Let sit at room temperature for 15 minutes, then cut the square bar in half, then cut crosswise into 1-inch-wide bars.

Store the bars in an airtight container in the freezer for up to 6 months.

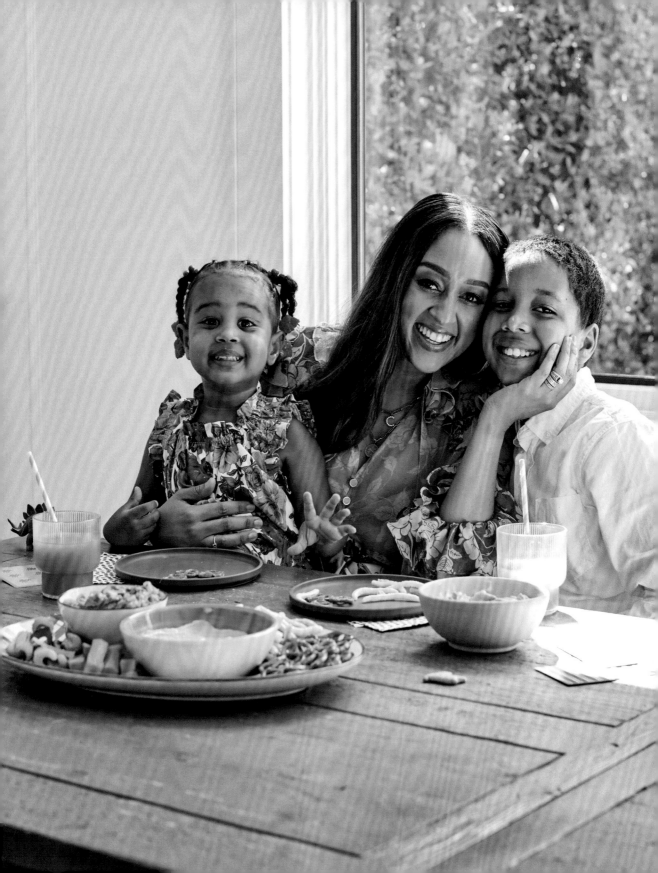

Snacks

Old-School Granola Bars

SERVES 6 TO 8

PREP TIME: 10 minutes

TOTAL TIME: 35 minutes

Nonstick cooking spray

1½ cups old-fashioned rolled oats

1 cup all-purpose flour

1 teaspoon baking soda

½ teaspoon kosher salt

1 large egg

½ cup creamy peanut butter
   or sunflower seed butter

⅓ cup honey

½ to ⅔ cup grape or strawberry
   jelly or jam (or whatever you
   have in your fridge!)

Tia's Tips

Don't shy away from this if your child is allergic to nuts. Sunflower butter works just as well.

To make this gluten-free, you can substitute any all-purpose gluten-free flour, and of course always read the label of the old-fashioned oats.

Remember when I said I hated when my PB&J sandwich got smashed on the bottom of my backpack? Here's the solution! A bite into this is a wave of nostalgia like no other, and I like making my own granola bars because I can control the sugar and eliminate the processing and additives. Because this is such a quick recipe (and because it's hands-on!), the kids enjoy helping out. These make a great midmorning snack or a filler-upper when Cree comes home from school.

Preheat the oven to 350°F. Line an 8 × 8-inch or 9 × 9-inch baking dish with parchment paper. Lightly spritz with cooking spray.

In a large bowl, mix the oats, flour, baking soda, and salt.

In another bowl, whisk together the egg, peanut butter, and honey. Whisk until fully mixed, pour over the bowl of oats, and fold until the oats are coated. Spread three-quarters of the mixture on the bottom of the pan, pressing into the corners. Make sure it is level, so it can cook evenly.

Top with jam or jelly and spread evenly. Sprinkle with the remaining oat mixture. Gently press down. Bake until the crust is golden brown, 25 to 30 minutes. Remove from the oven and let cool completely. For easier cutting, place the cooled pan in the refrigerator for 30 minutes. Remove the granola from the pan using parchment paper. Place on a cutting board and cut into bars.

Store in an airtight container in the refrigerator for up to 2 weeks.

Apple Donut Rings

SERVES 2 OR 3
PREP TIME: 5 minutes
TOTAL TIME: 5 minutes

1 apple, well washed and dried

Nut butter of your choice

TOPPINGS

Chopped nuts

Shredded coconut

Mini chocolate chips

Chocolate Cherry Granola
  (page 143)

Dried fruit

Ground cinnamon

Ground nutmeg

Oh, all right. You probably won't trick anyone into thinking these are actual donuts, but if you let your kids in on the process, they might just love them the same! I list suggested toppings here, but really, the possibilities are limitless. Close your eyes, imagine your favorite donut, and top accordingly.

Core the apple, then slice the apple crosswise into thin rings. Spread about 1 tablespoon nut butter on the top of an apple ring. Sprinkle with your favorite toppings. Serve immediately.

Tia's Tips

This is a great afternoon snack. Use apples with tartness, including Braeburn, Honeycrisp, Gala, Fuji, or Granny Smith. You can also use other fruits like pears and bananas, sliced lengthwise to create a longer surface for toppings.

If you don't have an apple corer, cut the apple into rings first, then use a knife to cut a circle around the seeds.

Mini Quesadilla Pizza

SERVES 1

PREP TIME: 5 minutes

TOTAL TIME: 10 minutes

½ tablespoon extra-virgin olive oil

2 (6-inch) tortillas, flour or corn

Shredded reduced-fat
    mozzarella cheese

Store-bought tomato sauce
    or BBQ sauce

FILLINGS AND/ OR TOPPINGS

Pepperoni slices

Crumbled cooked sausage

Mashed meatballs

Sliced olives

Cooked spinach

Cooked veggies

When pizza dough isn't around, this is a great alternative and everyone can build their own. When it comes to pizza, toppings are everything, so use the tortillas as a playground: Go crazy for meat lovers, sneak in vegetables for the kids, and get down! The fillings and toppings are interchangeable in this recipe.

In a skillet with a lid, heat the oil over medium heat until hot. Add a tortilla, sprinkle with some mozzarella cheese, and top with any filling you'd like. Cover with the second tortilla and cook until the bottom tortilla is golden brown and the edges are crispy, a few minutes.

Flip the quesadilla and spoon 2 tablespoons tomato sauce or BBQ sauce on top. Add your favorite toppings, then sprinkle with more mozzarella on top. Reduce the heat to medium-low and cover with the lid for a few minutes—this will help to melt the cheese. Remove to plate, cut, and serve.

Tia's Tips

Don't have tortillas? Use pitas or naan! Just slice in half and stuff with cheese and veggies.

If your kids are too young to use the stovetop, you can easily make this in a microwave or oven. Just fill, top, and warm until the cheese is melted.

Chocolate Chip Protein Bites

MAKES 18 BITES; SERVES 6

PREP TIME: 15 minutes

TOTAL TIME: 15 minutes

1 cup old-fashioned rolled oats

½ cup nut butter

½ cup ground flaxseeds, hemp hearts, or chia seeds

½ cup mini chocolate chips or raisins

¼ cup honey, maple syrup, or agave nectar

¼ teaspoon kosher salt

2 scoops protein powder or collagen (optional)

What I love about these is the combo of healthy good fats and carbs to keep you, the kids, the hubby, the friends (whomever!) fuller longer. These will help the between-meal moments of the day without spoiling that precious and patient appetite.

In a large bowl, mix together the oats, nut butter, flaxseeds, chocolate chips, honey, salt, and protein powder (if using).

Using a 1-tablespoon ice cream scoop, scoop heaping portions onto a parchment-lined sheet pan (you should get about 18). With clean hands, roll into smooth balls. Eat right away or place in the refrigerator for 30 minutes.

Store in an airtight container for a week or freeze for 3 months.

Tia's Tip

If you are using protein powder and it is sweetened, you may need to reduce the honey.

Variation

Experiment with other ingredients, like dried fruits or chopped nuts instead of chocolate chips. Or, if you want it to be rich and chocolaty, mix in ¼ cup unsweetened cacao powder.

Banana "Sushi" Rolls

SERVES 1
PREP TIME: 5 minutes
TOTAL TIME: 5 minutes

TOPPINGS

Shredded coconut

Mini chocolate chips

Chopped nuts of any kind

Freeze-dried raspberries,
strawberries, or blueberries

Thinly sliced fresh strawberries

Dried cranberries

Sprinkles

"SUSHI" ROLLS

1 (6-inch) flour tortilla

1 tablespoon nut butter,
plus more for sealing
and topping

1 medium banana, peeled
but whole

Who knows, maybe this is the gateway snack that familiarizes your kids with sushi. Or maybe it's just a delightful new take on bananas that gives in to your sweet tooth. Call the kids over for this one, but if you're not comfy with them cutting, leave the roll whole to eat like a burrito.

Place all the toppings in small bowls or plates.

MAKE THE "SUSHI" ROLLS: Lay the tortilla on the cutting board. Thinly and evenly spread the nut butter to cover the entire tortilla. Place the whole banana on the lower part of the tortilla. Roll the tortilla tightly. Use more nut butter if needed to make sure the tortilla stays closed.

Spread a very thin layer of nut butter over the rolled tortilla. Slice the roll crosswise into 1-inch discs. Dip the tortilla disc into your favorite toppings. Place on a plate and serve immediately.

Tia's Tips

This can't be stored because the banana begins to brown and get mushy, so make sure to serve and nibble right away.

If your kids are allergic to nuts, substitute sunflower butter or jam on the tortilla.

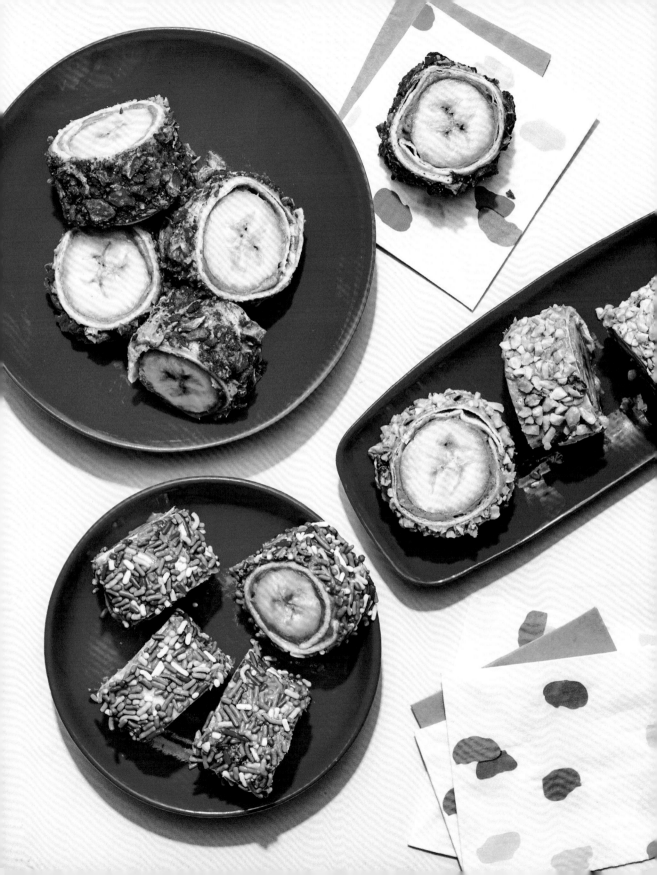

Tia's Tip

Another "blank canvas" bean is chickpeas! Got those in your pantry? Give them a whirl in this recipe.

Apple Pie Dip

MAKES 2 CUPS

PREP TIME: 5 minutes

TOTAL TIME: 10 minutes

⅔ cup unsweetened applesauce

1 (15-ounce) can white beans, rinsed and drained

1 tablespoon fresh lemon juice

¼ cup nut butter or tahini

¼ cup honey, plus more as needed

1 teaspoon ground cinnamon

½ teaspoon ground nutmeg

⅛ teaspoon chili powder (optional)

Pinch of kosher salt

Dippers (pretzels, pita chips, animal crackers, celery sticks, apples slices, cucumber slices, or carrot sticks), for serving

Yup! I'm using white beans for a sweet snack. Don't knock it 'til you try it! You'll be surprised to find that beans make a wonderful blank canvas for savory or sweet foods. Although you can pair just about anything with this tasty dip, I love pretzels. Something about that marriage of sweet and salty gets me *every* time.

Line a bowl with paper towels. Add the applesauce and allow the paper towels to absorb some of the liquid of the applesauce.

Scrape the applesauce into a food processor and add the beans, lemon juice, nut butter, honey, cinnamon, nutmeg, chili powder (if using), and salt. Process until smooth. Taste for seasoning and sweetness and add more honey if needed.

Serve with dippers. This recipe is good the same day, but the longer it sits in the refrigerator, the more the flavors blend together: The bean flavor lessens and the apple amplifies.

Store in the refrigerator in an airtight container for 1 week.

Variation

Make an edible, egg free chocolate chip cookie dough with this recipe by omitting the applesauce and lemon juice and adding ½ cup semisweet chocolate chips after the dip is blended smoothly.

Bagel Poppers

**MAKES 10 BAGEL POPPERS;
SERVES 3 OR 4**

PREP TIME: 5 minutes

TOTAL TIME: 30 minutes

1 cup all-purpose flour, plus more
as needed

1½ teaspoons baking powder

1 teaspoon kosher salt

1 cup nonfat plain Greek yogurt

Bagel seasoning, such as dried
onion, sesame seeds,
or poppy seeds

The sky's the limit with these bagel bites. If you're having a playdate, place toppings in bowls and have the kids decorate their own. They're also a perfect Sunday football snack if you're watching the morning games.

Position a rack in the center of the oven and preheat the oven to 375°F. Line a sheet pan with parchment paper.

In a medium bowl, whisk together the flour, baking powder, and salt. Add the yogurt. Using a wooden spoon or rubber spatula, combine until a dough forms and begins to pull away from the sides. If the dough seems wet, add a little flour 1 tablespoon at a time.

With a small ice cream scoop, scoop about 1 tablespoon of dough onto the lined sheet pan, spacing the scoops 1 to 2 inches apart. Sprinkle generously with your chosen bagel seasoning.

Transfer to the oven and bake until deep golden brown, 25 to 30 minutes, rotating the pan front to back halfway through.

Store in an airtight container at room temperature for 4 days (if your family doesn't eat them up before then!). You can reheat if desired.

Variations

Love garlic knots? Top with garlic salt and melted butter!

Want sweet? After the dough is mixed, stir in ½ cup raisins and 1 teaspoon ground cinnamon for a raisin bagel.

Tia's Tip

Embrace your favorite bagel! Use the typical minced dried onions, sesame seeds, poppy seeds, or salt. Or go to your local bagel shop and scan the varieties to inspire you.

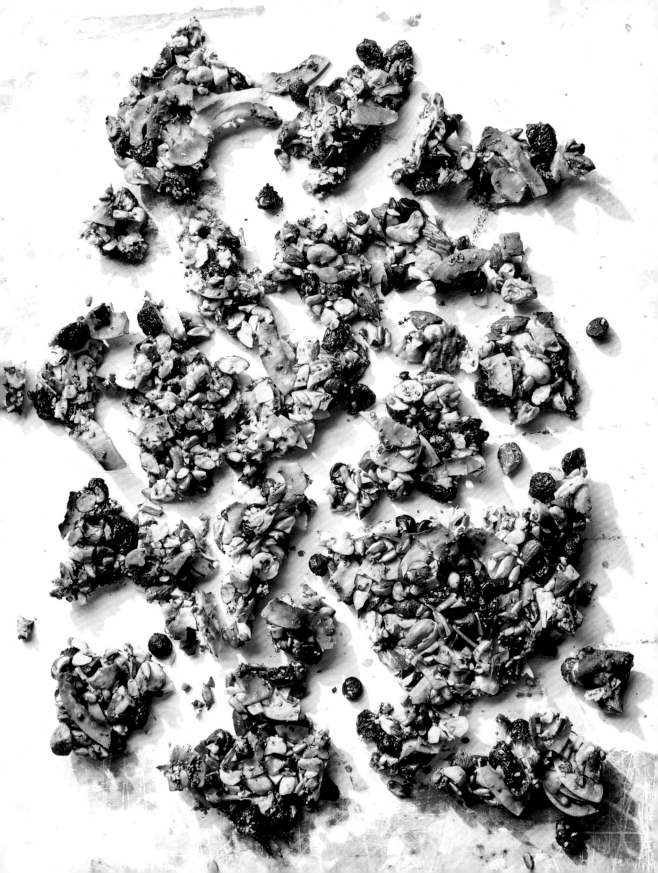

Trail Mix Bark

SERVES 6

PREP TIME: 10 minutes

TOTAL TIME: 1 hour 45 minutes

2 cups assorted raw nuts, coarsely chopped

½ cup unsweetened coconut flakes

¼ cup dried cranberries or raisins

¼ cup sunflower seeds

¼ cup semisweet chocolate chips

1 tablespoon chia seeds (optional)

¼ teaspoon fine sea salt

2 egg whites

¼ cup maple syrup or honey

Tia's Tips

If the bars are still sticky after cooling, you may need to bake them a few minutes longer next time to better caramelize the maple syrup.

This recipe works flawlessly when doubled, so do your future self a favor by making extra! Freeze half for quick grab-and-go action at a later date. You'll thank yourself!

Is this candy or is it a healthy snack? Is it dessert or is it the protein-packed yummy I bring on a hike? I'll tell you what it is, it's one of my favorite morsels of guilt-free pleasures ever. And those chia seeds will give you a hearty dose of daily fiber we all need to maintain productive digestion and a healthy microbiome. This treat is so delicious you won't know it's good for you!

Position a rack in the center of the oven and preheat the oven to 325°F. Line a sheet pan with parchment paper.

In a large bowl, combine the nuts, coconuts flakes, cranberries, sunflower seeds, chocolate chips, chia seeds (if using), and salt and stir until combined. In a small bowl, whisk the egg whites and maple syrup until frothy. Pour over the nut mixture and toss until all the nuts are coated. Spread onto the lined sheet pan and use clean hands or a rubber spatula to push the mixture together and flatten, trying not to leave any gaps in the nut mixture.

Transfer to the oven and bake until the nuts are slightly darker, 30 to 35 minutes, rotating the pan front to back halfway through. Remove from the oven and let cool completely on the pan, about 1 hour.

Once cooled, use clean hands to break the bark into pieces.

Store in airtight containers with a sheet of parchment paper in between layers to prevent them from sticking together. These will keep for up to 1 week in the fridge or 2 months in the freezer. If frozen, let them thaw at room temperature for 15 to 20 minutes before eating.

Homemade Cheese(It) Crackers

SERVES 2

PREP TIME: 5 minutes

TOTAL TIME: 25 minutes

10 slices sharp cheddar cheese

Garlic salt

I have a friend who puts Goldfish crackers in her salads. At first, I couldn't quite wrap my head around it, but when I tried it . . . MIND BLOWN. With these, either eat them as crackers, or do as she does by adding a surprise to your plate of greens! Or pump up burgers or tacos with them. Truly, anything you put cheese on, sub in these cheesy crackers. It's the cheese you love, but crunchy!

Preheat the oven to 350°F. Line a sheet pan with parchment paper.

Stack all the cheese slices on top of each other, then cut into quarter squares. Separate into individual mini-squares and arrange on the lined pan about 2 inches apart. Sprinkle each square with a pinch of garlic salt.

Bake until the cheese has melted but the crackers still retain a square-ish shape, about 15 minutes. Remove from the oven and let cool for 5 minutes on the pan. The crackers will get crisper as they cool. Serve immediately.

Tia's Tips

Only use parchment paper for this recipe to ensure the crackers don't stick.

Sharp cheddar gives these crackers the intense cheese flavor, but other cheeses, such as Monterey Jack, Havarti, and provolone, also work. But for different cheeses you may need to increase the cook time by 1 minute.

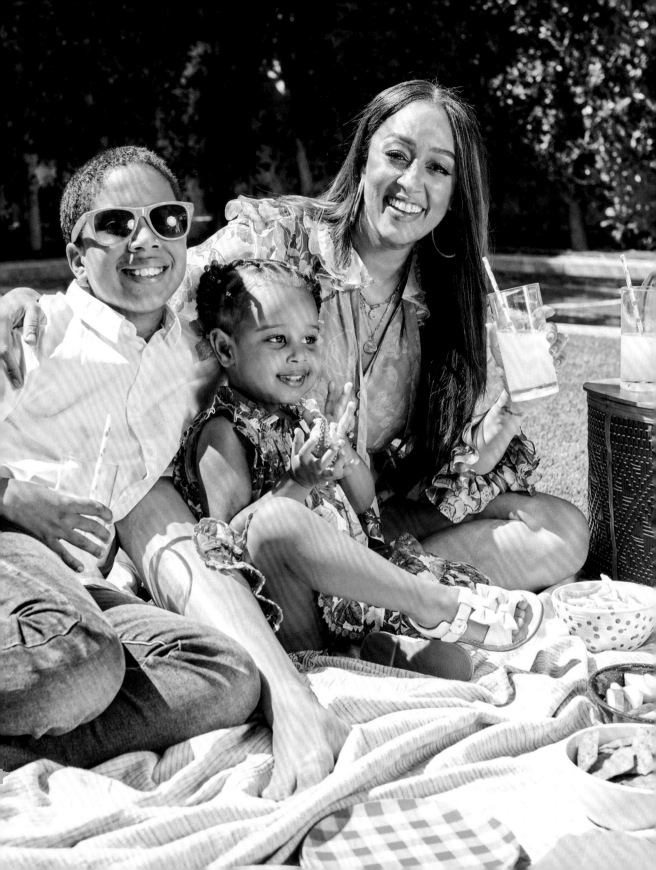

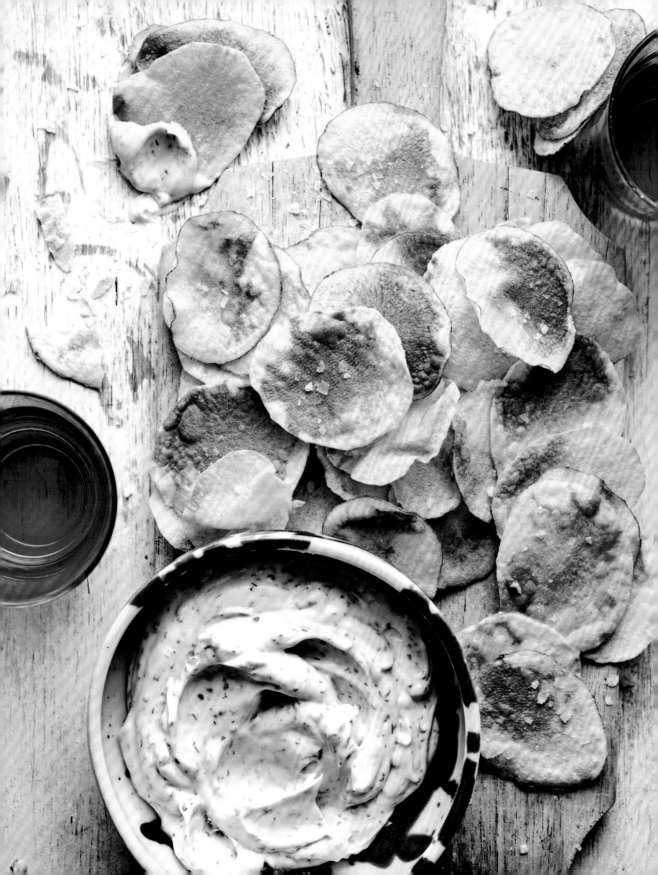

Quick Ranch Dip
& Homemade Potato Chips

SERVES 4

PREP TIME: 15 minutes

TOTAL TIME: 20 minutes

QUICK RANCH DIP

1½ cups mayonnaise

1 teaspoon apple cider vinegar or distilled white vinegar

1 teaspoon dried dill

1 teaspoon dried parsley

1 teaspoon garlic powder

1 teaspoon onion powder

Kosher salt and freshly ground black pepper

HOMEMADE POTATO CHIPS

1 medium potato, peeled

Olive oil cooking spray

2 teaspoons kosher salt

Tia's Tips

This ranch dip is also great as a salad dressing, a dip for chicken wings, or tossed with cold pasta. If using for a salad dressing, thin it out by whisking in ¼ cup milk of choice. Refrigerate for at least 1 hour before serving or overnight.

Chips: The water bath helps to remove the starch in potatoes and create crispy chips, so don't skip this step.

Ain't no shame in craving potato chips and dip. Believe me, it's difficult to resist when there's a bowl in front of me. But rather than buying a bag with all the processed gunk, I make them myself. Once you get the hang of the ranch recipe, it's easy to play with the spices to tailor to your palate. Dried spices and herbs are amazing for a quick recipe like this.

MAKE THE QUICK RANCH DIP: In a medium bowl, mix together the mayonnaise, vinegar, dill, parsley, garlic powder, and onion powder until fully combined. Season with salt and pepper to taste. Store in the refrigerator for 1 week in an airtight container.

MAKE THE HOMEMADE POTATO CHIPS: Fill a large bowl three-quarters full with water and 1 cup ice. Thinly slice the potato. The thinner the better, about ⅛ inch thick. Place the slices in the ice water and stir for 2 to 3 minutes to release some of the starch.

Drain the potatoes and dry both sides of the slices, by patting dry with paper towels—the dryer the better. Line a microwave-safe plate with parchment paper. Lay the slices on the plate without the slices touching. Spritz with the cooking spray and sprinkle with the salt. All microwaves are not created equal, so start microwaving on high for roughly 2 minutes 30 seconds to 3 minutes 30 seconds on one side. Flip and cook until golden brown and crispy, another 2 to 3 minutes. Be careful—the plate will be hot. Eat immediately. Repeat with any remaining potato slices.

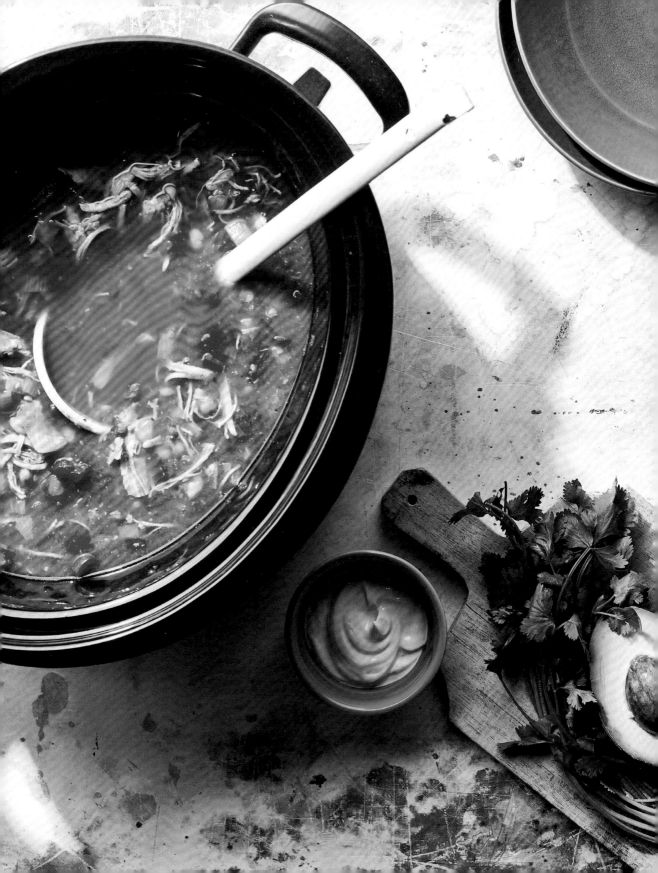

One-Pot & Sheet-Pan Wonders

Veggie Tamale Pie

SERVES 6 TO 8
PREP TIME: 20 minutes
TOTAL TIME: 1 hour

ENCHILADA SAUCE

4½ cups water

2 (6-ounce) cans tomato paste

⅓ cup reduced-sodium
  soy sauce or tamari

¼ cup honey

Half a 1-ounce packet
  taco seasoning

½ teaspoon freshly ground
  black pepper

TAMALE PIE

3 tablespoons extra-virgin oil

2 (1-pound) tubes premade
  polenta

3 cups corn tortilla chips,
  lightly crushed

2 medium zucchini, cut into
  ¼-inch dice

1 red bell pepper, cut into
  ¼-inch dice

1 bunch scallions, finely chopped

Half a 1-ounce packet
  taco seasoning

1 teaspoon kosher salt

½ teaspoon freshly ground
  black pepper

3 cups shredded cheddar cheese

6 (6-inch) corn tortillas

In this dish, you'll experience three different types of corn, giving your mouth a roller coaster of texture: creamy, crunchy, and chewy. When cooking dinners like this, I often add an element that is already made, which REALLY saves on time and energy. Here, I grab premade polenta from the pasta section of the store (it comes in a tube shape), use taco seasoning rather than rounding up half the pantry's spices to make my own, and assign Cairo the job of crumbling the tortilla chips and pressing down the polenta. It's like she's shaping Play-Doh!

Preheat the oven to 400°F.

MAKE THE ENCHILADA SAUCE: In a blender, combine the water, tomato paste, soy sauce, honey, taco seasoning, and pepper. Blend until fully combined. Set aside.

ASSEMBLE THE TAMALE PIE: Grease a 9 × 13-inch baking dish with 1 tablespoon of the oil. Using a fork or clean hands, press the polenta into the bottom of the baking dish until it is covered completely. Sprinkle the crushed chips over the polenta. Pour 2 cups of the enchilada sauce over the chips. Add the zucchini, bell pepper, and scallions and spread to cover. Drizzle with the remaining 2 tablespoons oil and evenly sprinkle with the taco seasoning, salt, and pepper. Sprinkle with 1 cup of the cheddar. Lay the tortillas on top of the cheese, overlapping. Spread 1 cup of the enchilada sauce to cover the tortillas, then carefully flip over the tortillas and coat the other side with the remaining sauce.

RECIPE + INGREDIENTS CONTINUE

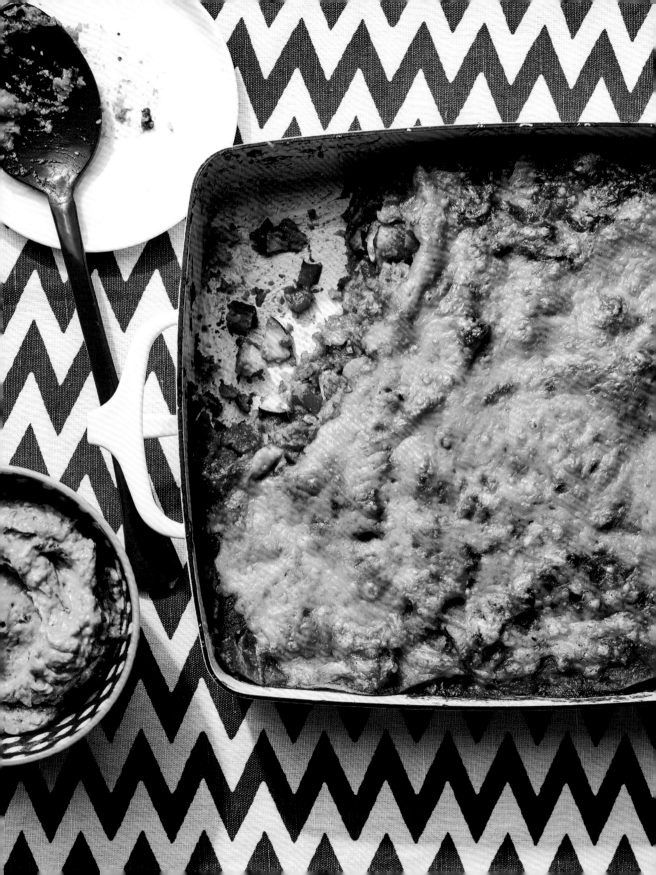

OPTIONAL TOPPINGS

Salsa

Sour cream

Guacamole

Cover with foil and bake until the sauce is bubbling, 30 to 35 minutes. Remove the foil and sprinkle the remaining 2 cups cheddar on top. Return to the oven to melt the cheese for 3 to 4 minutes.

Remove from the oven and let sit for 5 minutes before serving. Serve topped with salsa, sour cream, and/or guacamole.

Tia's Tip

In dishes like this I cut the veggies small, otherwise they might not cook through all the way.

Cheeseburger Soup

Hold the Bun

SERVES 4

PREP TIME: 15 minutes

TOTAL TIME: 30 minutes

3 tablespoons extra-virgin olive oil

1 medium yellow onion, diced

1 (14.5-ounce) can diced tomatoes, undrained

1 pound ground beef or ground turkey (93% lean)

1 teaspoon garlic salt

1 tablespoon spicy brown mustard

1 large russet or 2 medium Yukon Gold potatoes, peeled and diced

4 cups reduced-sodium beef or chicken broth

¼ cup chopped dill pickles (about 1 large)

1 teaspoon dried parsley

1½ cups shredded sharp cheddar cheese or ⅓ cup nutritional yeast

1½ cups half-and-half or 1 (13.5-ounce) can coconut milk

1 tablespoon cornstarch

¼ cup water

Kosher salt and freshly ground black pepper

I mean, who doesn't love a burger? And who doesn't love soup? Good thing I found a way to combine both for you into one pot! You are very welcome.

In a large deep skillet or soup pot, heat the oil over medium-high heat. Add the onion and sauté until soft, about 5 minutes. Add the tomatoes and their juices, increase the heat to high, and cook until most of the liquid has evaporated. Add the beef and garlic salt and brown until the meat is no longer pink. Stir in the mustard until fully combined. Add the potatoes, beef broth, chopped pickles, and dried parsley.

Bring to a simmer and cook, uncovered, until the potatoes are tender, 8 to 10 minutes. Add the cheddar (or nutritional yeast, if using) and half-and-half (or coconut milk, if using) and stir until the cheese has melted. Let simmer for another 5 minutes, uncovered.

In a small bowl, whisk together the cornstarch and water. Add to the soup, bring to a boil, and allow the soup to thicken for a few minutes. Season with salt and pepper to taste and serve.

Tia's Tips

Both dairy and nondairy options are equally delicious here. Coconut milk adds a "Mmm, what's that?" nuance to the soup without bringing an overpowering coconut flavor.

Cornstarch whisked into water is called a "slurry," which thickens sauces, gravies, and soups. You'll see this technique a few times in the recipes.

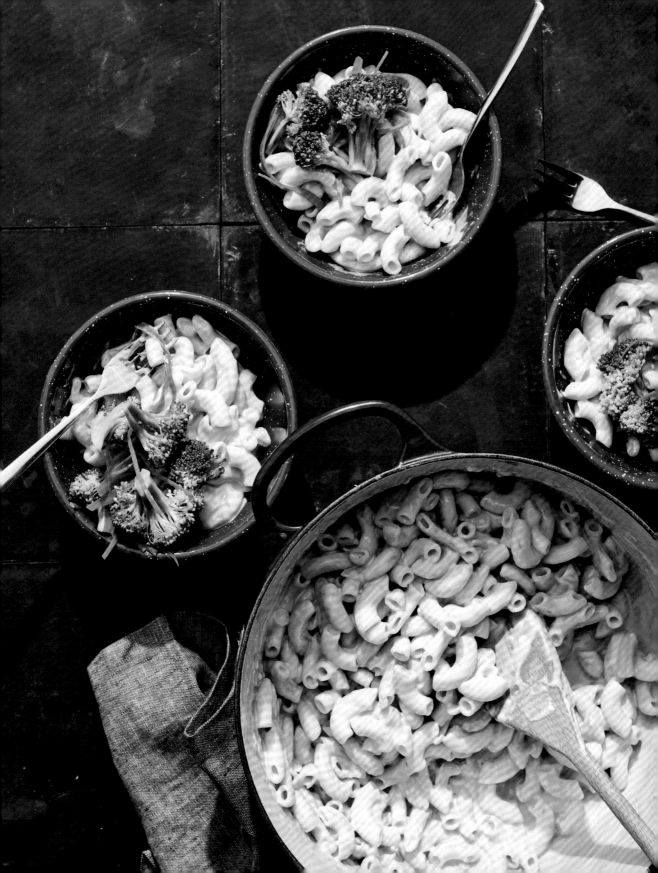

Creamy Mac & Cheese

SERVES 4 OR 5

PREP TIME: 20 minutes

TOTAL TIME: 40 minutes

MAC AND CHEESE

3 tablespoons unsalted butter

1 pound elbow macaroni or small shells

4 cups milk, unsweetened nondairy milk, chicken stock, or vegetable stock

1 cup shredded sharp cheddar cheese or a blend

1 teaspoon kosher salt

1 teaspoon garlic powder

SAUTÉED BROCCOLI

1 tablespoon olive oil or avocado oil

2 cups bite-size broccoli florets

1 cup shredded carrots

Kosher salt or bagel seasoning

Tia's Tips

You can buy preshredded carrots or take whole carrots, scrub them (no peeling necessary), and grate with a box grater.

Cutting vegetables smaller helps them cook in this method.

Nope, mac and cheese does *not* need to be baked! Nor does it absolutely need milk to create that sumptuous velvet coating on the noodles. Here, I use a risotto technique—gradually incorporating liquid until the pasta is cooked—which brings out the starches and creates a natural creamy texture. Of course, you can still use milk for added richness, but broth works well and also gives the mac depth of flavor. I've also added sautéed broccoli for a healthy veggie!

MAKE THE MAC AND CHEESE: In a large skillet, melt the butter over medium heat. Stir in the pasta and ½ cup of the milk (or other liquid) and stir constantly until the liquid is absorbed. Continue adding liquid ½ cup at a time, allowing the liquid to absorb each time before adding the next amount, until the pasta is tender, 20 to 25 minutes. Once the pasta is cooked, remove from the heat, add the cheese, salt, and garlic powder. Stir until the cheese is melted. If the pasta looks dry, add a bit more liquid.

SAUTÉ THE BROCCOLI: In a medium skillet, heat the oil over medium-high heat. Add the broccoli and carrots and cook, stirring, until the broccoli becomes a bright green, 3 to 5 minutes. Add a few tablespoons water to the pan and swirl the pan. Let the water steam and evaporate. Sprinkle with salt to taste. If you have a picky eater, try using bagel seasoning, just omit the salt.

Divide the mac and cheese into bowls, add the broccoli on top, and serve. You can also plate the broccoli separately as a side dish!

Shrimp & Pork Fried Rice

SERVES 4
PREP TIME: 15 minutes
TOTAL TIME: 35 minutes

6 slices bacon, cut crosswise into ½-inch strips

2 tablespoons neutral oil (canola or grapeseed oil)

6 garlic cloves, coarsely chopped

2 large shallots, diced

1 pound medium shrimp, peeled, deveined, and tail removed

4 cups cooked rice

2 tablespoons fish sauce

2 tablespoons hoisin sauce

2 tablespoons reduced-sodium soy sauce

1 teaspoon chili-garlic sauce, or more to taste

1 teaspoon ground ginger

1 teaspoon kosher salt, plus more to taste

1 teaspoon freshly ground black pepper, plus more to taste

2 cups frozen vegetables (peas, carrots, corn, etc.)

2 cups snow peas (optional)

On Rachael Ray's old show, she used to walk to her pantry with an empty bowl and fill it up with the ingredients she needed. Sometimes if a bowl wasn't enough, she put the bowl on a baking sheet and stacked everything in the bowl and then on the baking sheet until it almost covered her eyes. Still makes me laugh! She would do anything to avoid more than one trip around the kitchen. This is a good recipe to try out one-trip skills. Grab a vessel, walk on over to your pantry, and fill 'er up with the goodness fried rice brings.

In a large skillet, cook the bacon over medium-high heat until crispy. Remove to a paper plate lined with paper towels.

Add the oil to the bacon fat in the skillet and stir in the garlic and shallots. Cook over medium-high heat until soft, 3 to 5 minutes, being careful not to burn the garlic. Add the shrimp and sauté until they turn pink, about 2 minutes. Toss in the rice and coat with the fat in the pan. Stir in the fish sauce, hoisin sauce, soy sauce, chili-garlic sauce, ginger, salt, and pepper. Cook the rice for 1 to 2 more minutes, folding constantly and mixing all the ingredients well.

Add the frozen vegetables and snow peas (if using). Allow the heat of the rice to cook them for 3 to 5 minutes. Taste for more salt and pepper. Serve while warm. This makes great leftovers for the next day, if there is any left.

Tia's Tips

Day-old rice or frozen cooked rice works in this recipe because it has less moisture and can crisp up a bit. However, if you don't have it, just cook your rice as normal and use that. If you eat a lot of rice, make it in big batches, let it cool completely, and freeze it in family-size portions. Then microwave when ready to eat.

The chili-garlic sauce in this recipe balances the sweet and sour but it's not quite enough to make it spicy. If you add more, then get ready for the heat. So, start with 1 teaspoon and keep adding until your heart's content.

Snow peas are added at the end and slightly cook with the heat of the rice and pan. They keep crisp and bright green. If you like them cooked more, blanch before adding.

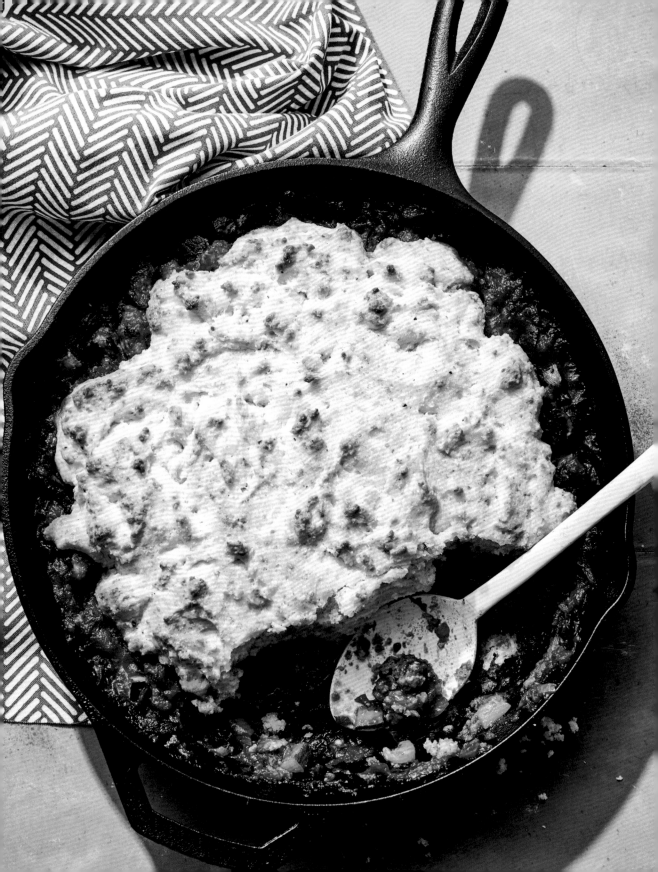

Italian Pot Pie

SERVES 6 TO 8

PREP TIME: 20 minutes

TOTAL TIME: 40 minutes

1 pound bulk sweet
Italian sausage

4 tablespoons extra-virgin
olive oil

8 ounces sliced mushrooms

1 medium zucchini, cut into
½-inch cubes

1 green bell pepper, grated
or finely chopped

1 small yellow onion, grated
or finely chopped

1 (28-ounce) can crushed
tomatoes

3 garlic cloves, grated or minced

1 teaspoon dried oregano

1 teaspoon kosher salt

½ teaspoon freshly ground
black pepper

TOPPING

2 cups all-purpose flour

½ cup grated parmesan cheese

1 tablespoon baking powder

½ teaspoon dried oregano

½ teaspoon kosher salt

½ teaspoon freshly ground
black pepper

1½ cups milk

½ cup (1 stick) unsalted butter,
melted

This is not your grandmother's pot pie. Rather, it's that sweet grandma in Tuscany who discovered pot pies on her trip to America and wanted to reinvent them with Italian flair. The hearty vegetable sauce brings the comfort of the ol' pot pie with new flavors you'll enjoy. The mere size of this meal is great for crowds or a multinight leftover feast.

Preheat the oven to 400°F.

In a 10- or 12-inch cast-iron or ovenproof skillet, brown the sausage over medium heat, until it is no longer pink, about 7 minutes. Remove to a plate.

Add 2 tablespoons of the oil to the skillet and add the mushrooms in a single layer. Let cook without turning for a couple of minutes until browned. Stir in the zucchini and sauté until slightly browned and soft, about 5 minutes. Remove to the same plate as the sausage.

Add the remaining 2 tablespoons oil to the pan, then add the bell pepper and onion and sauté over medium high heat until soft, 3 to 5 minutes.

Add the canned tomatoes, garlic, oregano, salt, and pepper. Return the sausage and vegetables to the pan and stir until combined. Reduce the heat to medium and simmer for 5 to 8 minutes, stirring occasionally.

RECIPE CONTINUES

MEANWHILE, MAKE THE TOPPING: In a medium bowl, whisk together the flour, parmesan, baking powder, oregano, salt, and pepper. Make a well in the center of the bowl and add the milk and melted butter. Stir until the batter is fully mixed; it should be slightly thicker than pancake batter. Don't overmix.

Remove the skillet from the heat and pour the batter evenly on top of the sauce, leaving a 1-inch border uncovered around the outsides of the pan. Transfer to the oven and bake until the mixture is bubbling and the crust is firm to the touch, 20 to 25 minutes. Turn the oven to broil and brown the top for a few minutes. Remove from the oven and let sit for 5 minutes before serving.

Store leftovers in an airtight container in the refrigerator for 5 to 6 days.

Tia's Tips

This recipe can be made with ground beef or turkey, or a combination of both. You can also substitute other vegetables like spinach or other leafy greens, and even yellow squash.

If you'd like to fancy it up, make individual servings by using ramekins and cooking for 15 minutes. These freeze well after baking, just let cool completely first.

Chicken Tortilla Soup

SERVES 5 OR 6

PREP TIME: 10 minutes

TOTAL TIME: 4 to 8 hours in a slow cooker; 5 to 8 minutes in a pressure cooker

1 red bell pepper,
    coarsely chopped

1 small yellow onion,
    coarsely chopped

1 (14.5-ounce) can diced tomatoes

4 cups low-sodium chicken stock

2 tablespoons tomato paste

2 teaspoons dried oregano

1 teaspoon garlic powder

1 teaspoon kosher salt

½ teaspoon freshly ground
    black pepper

2 boneless, skinless chicken
    breasts (4 to 5 ounces each)

1 (15-ounce) can cannellini, white
    beans, or navy beans, rinsed
    and drained

½ cup shredded cheddar cheese

¼ cup chopped fresh cilantro
    (optional)

TOPPINGS

Cubed or sliced avocado

Shredded cheddar cheese

Crushed tortilla chips

Sour cream

Okay, so this is a *slow* recipe, but the time you'll actively work on it is quick. I like making this on a cold weekend because all day the house smells of yummy soup, and who doesn't want that? Using a slow cooker is a great way to cook perfectly tender chicken that absorbs the deep flavoring from the other ingredients. The beans act as a thickener and bring creaminess (plus some added protein). And are you often stuck with crumbled tortilla chips at the bottom of the bag? Well, here's how to use those stragglers: crunchy garnish!

In a slow cooker, combine the bell pepper, onion, tomatoes, stock, tomato paste, oregano, garlic powder, salt, and black pepper and stir until fully combined. Nestle the chicken breasts into the mixture. Cover and cook on high for 4 hours or on low for 8 hours.

When done, transfer the chicken to a cutting board and use forks to shred the meat. Set aside.

Add the beans to the slow cooker. Using an immersion blender, blend until almost smooth, but still a bit chunky. Add the shredded chicken and cheddar and stir until the cheese has melted. Stir in the cilantro (if using). Ladle into bowls and serve with toppings.

RECIPE CONTINUES

PRESSURE COOKER METHOD

Add the bell pepper, onion, tomatoes, stock, tomato paste, oregano, garlic powder, salt, and black pepper to the pot and stir until fully combined. Nestle the chicken breasts into the mixture. Cover and cook on high pressure for 5 minutes. Quick-release the pressure. Then follow the directions in the slow cooker version to finish, starting with shredding the chicken.

Tia's Tips

Do not remove the lid on the slow cooker until the end. I know it's tempting but it loses heat and takes more time to return to temperature.

If the liquid has reduced too much, add another cup of stock at the end of cooking.

If you do not have an immersion blender, carefully ladle some of the soup into a blender and blend until smooth. Be careful here, because the hot soup expands when blending and can burst out of the blender. Therefore, only fill about half full and remove the steam vent from the center of the blender lid. Return back to the slow cooker and stir.

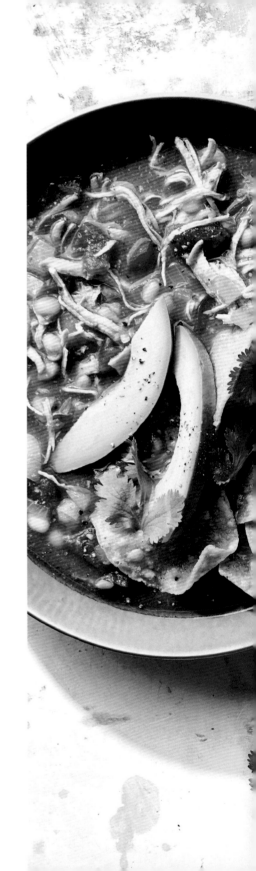

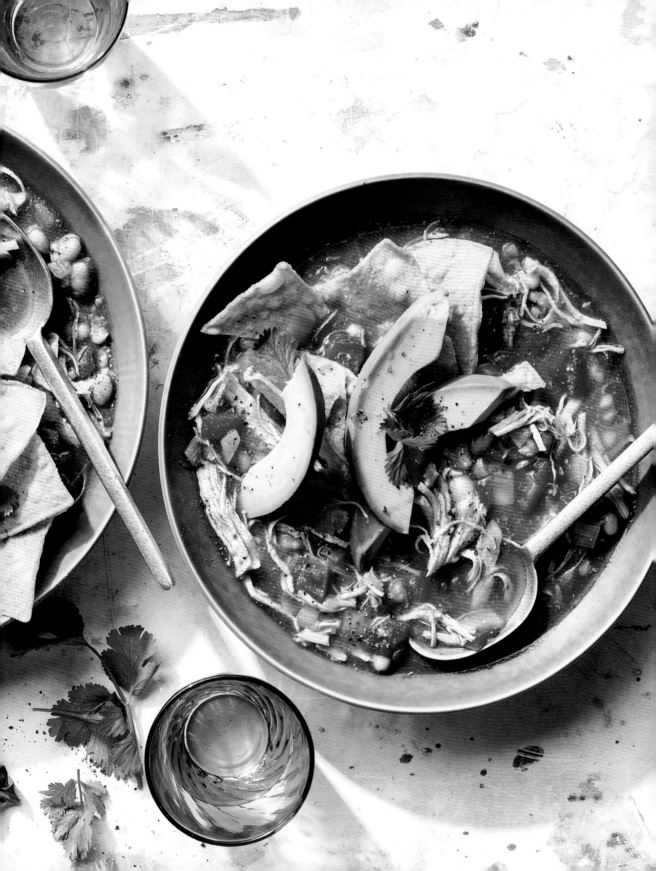

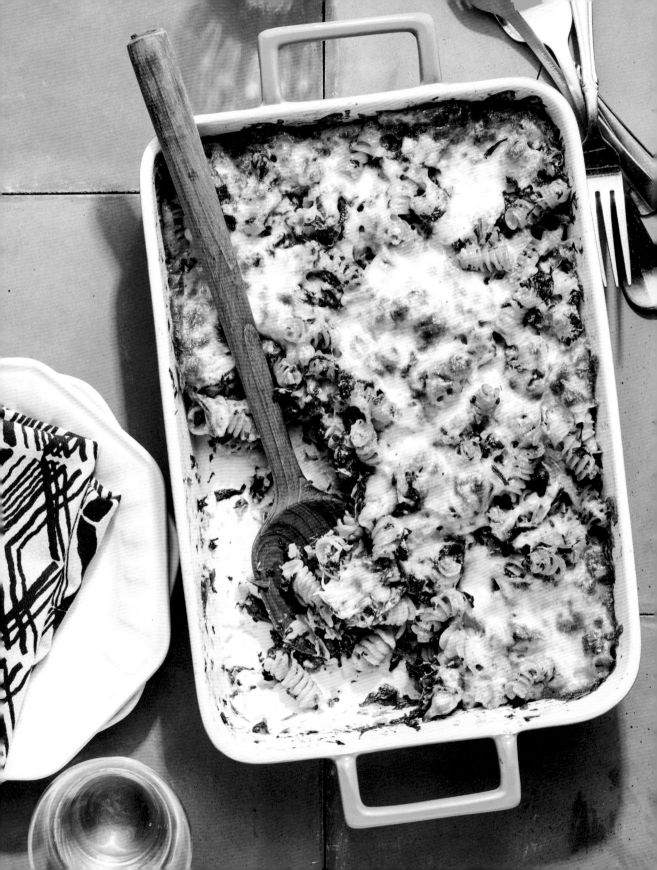

Spinach Artichoke Pasta Bake

SERVES 8 TO 10

PREP TIME: 20 minutes

TOTAL TIME: 55 minutes

Butter, for the baking dish

1 small yellow onion, grated

2 garlic cloves, minced or grated

1 pound penne or fusilli pasta

1 (12-ounce) container spinach artichoke dip

1½ cups shredded mozzarella cheese

1 (16-ounce) bag frozen baby spinach, thawed and squeezed dry

3 cups vegetable stock

½ cup grated parmesan cheese

Once I start with artichoke dip, I can't stop, especially when watching TV with a group of loved ones. So, why not translate that snack into a nighttime feast?

Preheat the oven to 350°F. Grease a 9 × 13-inch baking dish with butter.

Place the onion, garlic, pasta, dip, and ½ cup of the mozzarella in the prepared baking dish. If there are big chunks of spinach, break them with clean hands and add the spinach to the baking dish. Gently stir until everything is combined. Pour in the vegetable stock and stir until the pasta is coated with the artichoke mixture.

Cover with foil and bake for 30 to 35 minutes, stirring once or twice halfway through cooking. Remove the foil, sprinkle with the remaining 1 cup mozzarella and the parmesan, and bake until the cheese is melted and the pasta is cooked, another 5 to 10 minutes. Let sit for 5 minutes before serving.

This makes a lot of pasta leftovers. Store in an airtight container in the fridge for 5 to 6 days.

Tia's Tips

Stirring halfway through allows the pasta to cook evenly. If you don't stir, the top layer won't cook properly.

The big time-saver here is using frozen spinach. Otherwise, you would need to chop, cook, and drain off the liquid before adding.

Honey-Mustard Salmon with Asparagus & Butternut Squash

SERVES 4
PREP TIME: 10 minutes
TOTAL TIME: 30 minutes

Nonstick cooking spray

3 tablespoons extra-virgin olive oil

1 tablespoon Dijon or whole-grain mustard

1 tablespoon honey

½ teaspoon garlic powder

Kosher salt and freshly ground black pepper

4 (4-ounce) skin-on Atlantic salmon fillets

1 bunch thick asparagus, trimmed

Juice of ½ small lemon

3 cups ½-inch cubes butternut squash (about 2 pounds)

½ teaspoon chili powder

Salmon is a good starter fish for kids. It is light in flavor and doesn't have an overpowering ocean taste. Cooking it with a honey-mustard sauce refocuses the fishy taste, while adding a nice tangy zing. Use leftovers for a salmon salad. Cold salmon is delish!

Preheat the oven to 425°F. Lightly spritz the middle of a sheet pan with cooking spray.

In a small bowl, whisk together 1 tablespoon of the oil, the mustard, honey, garlic powder, and ½ teaspoon each salt and pepper.

Place the salmon in the middle of the prepared baking sheet, skin-side down. Drizzle the honey-mustard sauce on top and spread to cover all sides of the salmon. Add the asparagus to one side of the sheet pan. Drizzle the asparagus with 1 tablespoon of the oil and the lemon juice and sprinkle with ½ teaspoon each salt and pepper. Gently toss to coat. Add the butternut squash to the other side of the salmon. Drizzle with the remaining 1 tablespoon oil and sprinkle with ½ teaspoon each salt and pepper and the chili powder. Gently toss to coat.

RECIPE CONTINUES

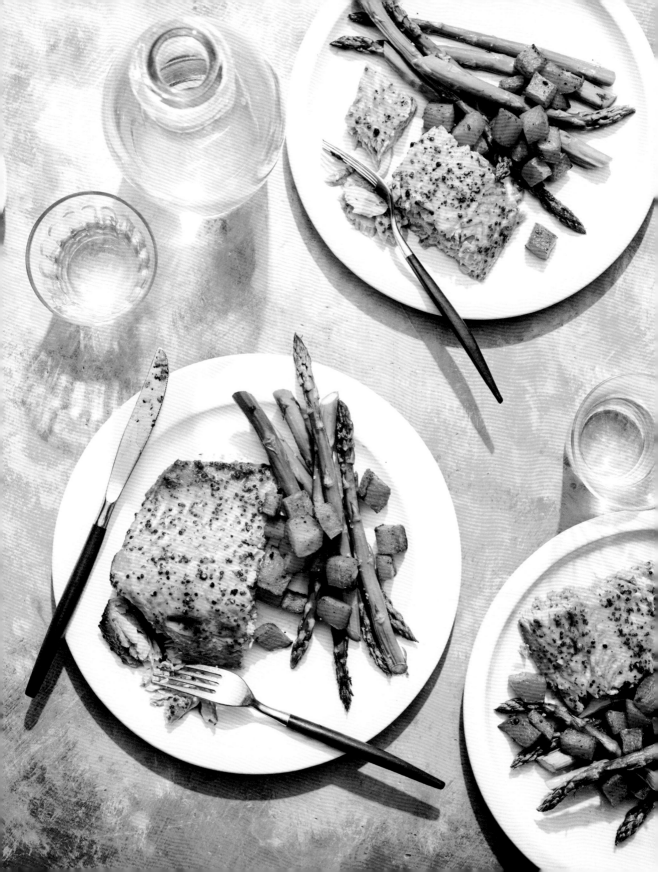

Bake until the squash is easily pierced with a knife and the salmon is cooked, 15 to 20 minutes. Serve hot.

Variations

No squash? Use sweet potato cubes.

Don't like asparagus? Try Brussels sprouts (cut in half) or green beans. Oven timing is about the same.

Tia's Tips

Okay, here's where precut veggies are essential: butternut squash. Like I said earlier, this is a tough vegetable to tackle unless you have a super-sharp knife and a very stable cutting board. Treat yourself if you can and have the work done for you. Otherwise, roast the whole butternut squash on a sheet pan lined with aluminum foil in a 300°F oven until just soft, 25 to 30 minutes. This makes cutting easier.

It's important that the squash is cut to the same size so everything cooks evenly. If the precut squash cubes you buy are a little bigger than ½ inch cubes, cut them down to size.

Chicken Fajita Tacos

SERVES 4 TO 6

PREP TIME: 10 minutes

TOTAL TIME: 40 minutes

FAJITAS

- 1 large yellow onion, cut into ¼-inch-wide slices
- 2 red bell peppers, cut in ¼-inch-wide strips
- 1 pint cherry tomatoes
- 2 ears corn, shucked
- 3 tablespoons extra-virgin olive oil
- 2 tablespoons Spice Rub (recipe follows)
- 2 boneless, skinless chicken breasts (6 ounces each)
- ½ teaspoon kosher salt
- 1 lime, halved
- Corn or flour tortillas
- ¼ cup chopped fresh cilantro leaves

FOR SERVING

- Shredded cheese
- Sour cream
- Guacamole
- Chopped cilantro

I cannot get enough of Mexican food, and luckily for me, I live in Los Angeles and have instant access to some of the best restaurants, food trucks, and taco stands in the world. Sometimes, though, I love filling my home with the smells and flavors of Mexican cuisine, and hearing that fajita sizzle in my own kitchen makes me want to dance. This one-pan version is a family favorite. And pssst . . . the baking sheet goes straight from the oven to the table. Voilà! One less dish to clean up.

Preheat the oven to 450°F.

PREPARE THE FAJITAS: Arrange the onion and bell peppers over three-quarters of the sheet pan. Add the cherry tomatoes and corn to the other side. Drizzle all the vegetables with 2 tablespoons of the oil, sprinkle with 1 tablespoon of the spice rub, and toss to coat. Place both chicken breasts on top of the onions and peppers. Drizzle the chicken with the remaining 1 tablespoon oil and sprinkle both sides of the chicken with the remaining 1 tablespoon spice rub. Season the entire pan with the salt. Place the lime halves, cut-side down, on the pan.

Transfer the pan to the oven and roast until the veggies are soft and the chicken is cooked through, 15 to 18 minutes. While the fajitas are cooking, wrap up the tortillas in foil and heat in the oven for 5 to 10 minutes.

RECIPE CONTINUES

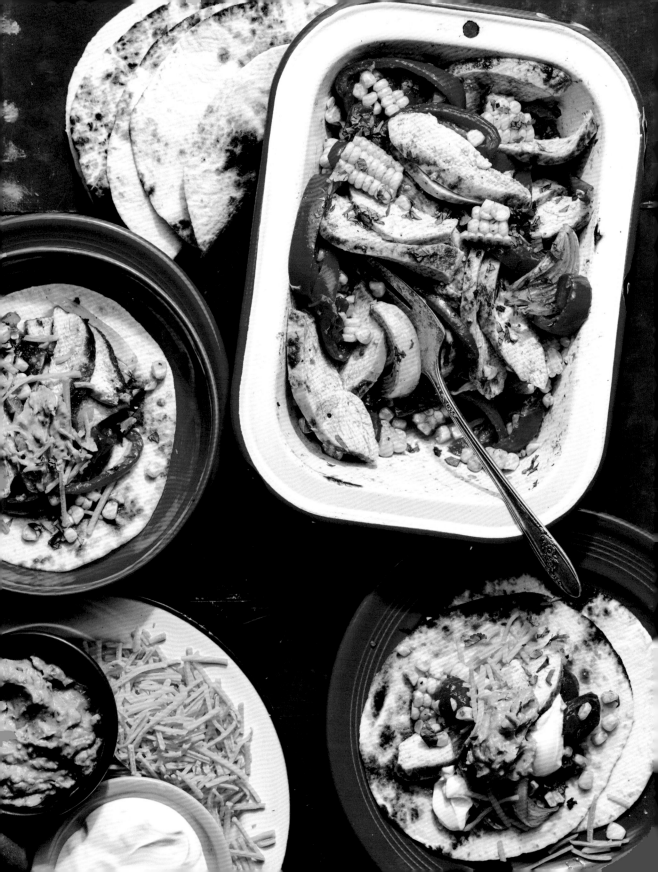

Tia's Tip

Rice and black beans are perfect side dishes. Add the spice rub to the beans and/or rice for a boost of flavor.

Remove everything from the oven. Place the chicken on a cutting board and let rest 5 minutes before cutting. Cut the kernels off the corn cobs. In a bowl, toss the corn with the roasted tomatoes. Sprinkle with the cilantro.

Slice the chicken into thin strips and return to the sheet pan. Squeeze the roasted lime halves over the entire pan.

TO SERVE: Set up a make-your-own bar and let everyone help themselves. Set out the chicken and vegetables, warmed tortillas, cheese, sour cream, guacamole, and cilantro.

Variation

Skirt steak will work for this dinner, too. It has the same cook time, but keep an eye on it.

SPICE RUB

MAKES 3 TABLESPOONS

1 tablespoon paprika

2 teaspoons kosher salt

1 teaspoon garlic powder

1 teaspoon onion powder

1 teaspoon ground coriander

1 teaspoon ground cumin

½ teaspoon freshly ground black pepper

In a medium bowl, mix the paprika, salt, garlic powder, onion powder, coriander, cumin, and black pepper. Store in an airtight container.

Beef, Broccoli & Rice

SERVES 6 TO 8
PREP TIME: 15 minutes
TOTAL TIME: 45 minutes

1½ cups medium-grain white rice

2½ cups low-sodium
   chicken broth

4 cups bite-size broccoli florets

1 large yellow onion, thinly sliced

2 green bell pepper, cut into
   ¼-inch-wide strips

1½ pounds skirt steak

1 teaspoon kosher salt

½ teaspoon freshly ground
   black pepper

SAUCE

2 garlic cloves, minced

½ cup reduced-sodium soy sauce

2 tablespoons balsamic vinegar

2 tablespoons light brown sugar

Pinch red pepper/chile flakes

1 teaspoon cornstarch

FOR SERVING

2 scallions, thinly sliced

1 tablespoon sesame seeds
   (optional)

Cooking this take-out favorite for yourself eliminates some of the unnatural additives that may be present at certain (but not all!) restaurants. It is delicious and cleanup is a breeze. And guess what, you throw the *uncooked* rice onto the sheet pan without the need to cook it separately.

Preheat the oven to 400°F.

Spread the rice evenly over a sheet pan. Pour the broth onto the rice and stir. Top with the broccoli, onion, and bell peppers. Set the skirt steak on top of the veggies and season both sides with the salt and pepper. Tightly cover the pan with foil and carefully transfer it to the oven. Cook until the rice and vegetables are tender, 30 to 35 minutes.

MEANWHILE, MAKE THE SAUCE: In a small saucepan, whisk together the garlic, soy sauce, vinegar, brown sugar, and chile flakes. Bring to a simmer over medium heat and cook for 5 minutes. In a small bowl, whisk the cornstarch and 2 tablespoons cold water until dissolved. Add the cornstarch mixture to the sauce and simmer until thickened. Remove from the heat and set aside.

Remove the sheet pan from the oven. Transfer the skirt steak to a cutting board and keep the foil over the broccoli and rice to keep it warm. Let the steak rest for 5 minutes before thinly slicing against the grain.

TO SERVE: Return the steak to the sheet pan and drizzle everything with the sauce. Sprinkle with the scallions and sesame seeds (if using) and gently toss and fluff with a fork. Serve while hot!

Tia's Tips

Since everything in the recipe cooks together, it is important to cut the veggies to the specific size indicated in the recipe.

Medium-grain rice is perfect for this cooking method.

Skirt steak is also called flap steak. It is thin with traces of fat throughout, great for quick cooking and flavor. If you can't find skirt, you can substitute a thin piece of flank steak.

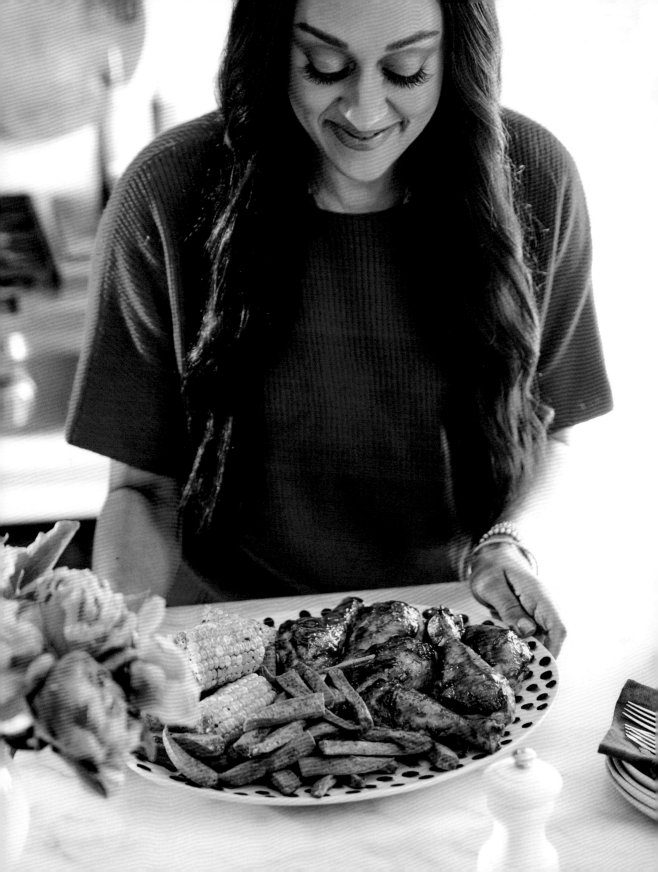

BBQ Chicken & Fries

SERVES 4

PREP TIME: 10 minutes

TOTAL TIME: 40 minutes

Nonstick cooking spray

6 chicken drumsticks
(about 4 ounces each)

1 cup store-bought barbecue
sauce, plus more (optional)
for serving

1 pound sweet potatoes (1 large
or 2 medium), peeled

4 ears corn, shucked and
cut in half

2 tablespoons extra-virgin
olive oil

1 teaspoon kosher salt

1 teaspoon paprika

½ teaspoon freshly ground
black pepper

Tia's Tips

Sometimes BBQ sauce has a little
too much spiciness for the kids.
A squirt of ketchup or honey tones
it down.

If drumsticks are not your favorite,
replace them with boneless,
skinless chicken thighs; just cook
both pans at the same time
for 20 to 30 minutes. Boneless
chicken thighs cooks faster than
drumsticks.

If it's raining or snowing outside and all you want is
something grilled, crank up the oven instead. This dish
brings the flavors you're craving and warms up the
house nicely.

Preheat the oven to 400°F. Line a sheet pan with foil and
lightly spritz a second pan with cooking spray.

Arrange the drumsticks on the foil-lined pan and generously
coat the chicken with ½ cup of the barbecue sauce. Bake for
10 minutes.

Meanwhile, cut the sweet potatoes into fries about ½ inch
thick. Arrange in a single layer on the sprayed pan. Add
the corn pieces to the pan. Drizzle everything with the oil
and sprinkle with the salt, paprika, and pepper. Using clean
hands, toss to coat.

Add the second sheet pan to the oven and remove the
pan with the drumsticks. Flip over the chicken and add the
remaining ½ cup barbecue sauce. Return to the oven.
Cook both pans until the chicken is no longer pink inside
and reaches an internal temperature of 175° to 180°F and the
sweet potatoes are tender, but charred around the edges,
another 20 to 30 minutes.

Remove the pans from the oven and drizzle the chicken with
more barbecue sauce, if desired. The heat of the chicken will
warm up the sauce. Serve immediately.

Stuffed Pesto Chicken Breast

SERVES 4

PREP TIME: 15 minutes

TOTAL TIME: 40 minutes

Nonstick cooking spray

4 ounces cold cream cheese

½ cup shredded
  mozzarella cheese

1½ tablespoons pesto,
  store-bought or homemade
  (see page 105)

1 large egg

1½ teaspoons kosher salt

½ cup shredded
  parmesan cheese

½ cup fine, dried bread crumbs,
  plain or Italian-style

4 boneless, skinless chicken
  breasts (about 4 ounces each)

2 medium zucchini, halved
  lengthwise and cut crosswise
  into ½-inch-thick half-moons

1 pint cherry tomatoes

2 tablespoons extra-virgin
  olive oil

½ teaspoon freshly ground
  black pepper

Cooked pasta, for serving
  (optional)

This one is definitely indulgent, and when we're eating it the table goes silent. All conversation hushes, and the only sounds are the enjoyment of each bite.

Preheat the oven to 400°F. Spritz a sheet pan with cooking spray.

In a small bowl, combine the cream cheese, mozzarella, and pesto. In a separate shallow bowl, whisk the egg and ½ teaspoon of the salt. On a flat plate, stir together the parmesan and bread crumbs.

Slice a horizontal pocket into each chicken breast; do not go all the way through. Stuff each pocket evenly with the pesto/cheese mixture.

Dip the stuffed chicken in the egg mixture, then coat both sides with parmesan bread crumbs. Place on the prepared sheet pan, leaving 2 inches space between the breasts. Arrange the zucchini and cherry tomatoes around the chicken. Drizzle with the oil and sprinkle with the remaining 1 teaspoon salt and the pepper. Using clean hands, gently toss the veggies to coat.

Bake until the chicken is cooked through, or until a thermometer inserted into the thickest part of the breast reads at least 165°F, 18 to 22 minutes. If the bread crumbs are starting to burn, lightly cover the chicken with foil. Remove from the oven and let rest for 5 minutes.

Serve the chicken with veggies on the side and/or a small portion of pasta, if desired.

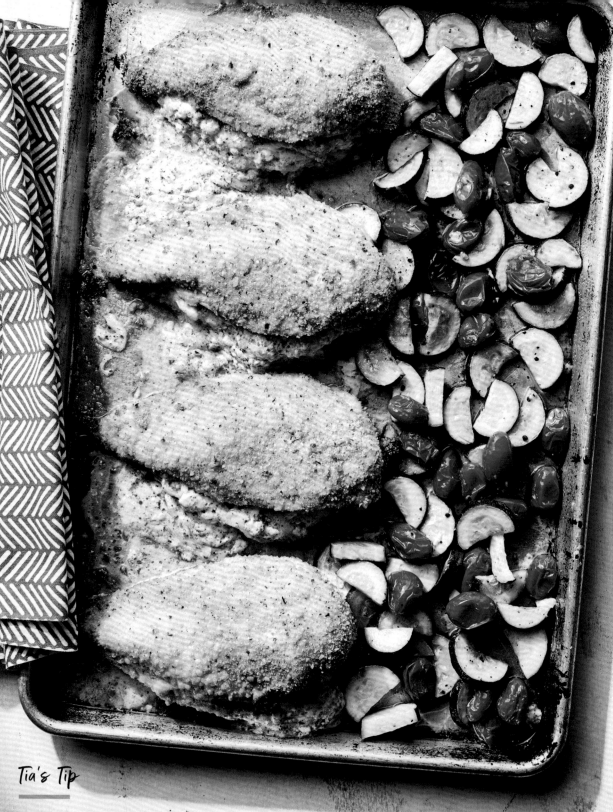

Tia's Tip

Keeping the cream cheese cold slows down the
melting process so it doesn't ooze out of the chicken.

Spatchcocked Lemon-Herb Chicken
with Roasted Baby Potatoes

SERVES 4
PREP TIME: 10 minutes
TOTAL TIME: 55 minutes

1 whole chicken (3 to 5 pounds)

2 lemons, thinly sliced

6 garlic cloves, smashed and peeled

Handful of fresh parsley, thyme, or cilantro

4 tablespoons (½ stick) unsalted butter, at room temperature

Kosher salt and freshly ground black pepper

2 pounds baby potatoes, rinsed and dried

2 tablespoons extra-virgin olive oil

1 tablespoon whole-grain mustard or spicy brown mustard

1 teaspoon ground cumin

If you love roasted chicken but want it faster, spatchcocking—removing the backbone and pressing down the chicken breast so it lies flat—is the way to go. It cooks evenly and more quickly, and by adding the aromatics under the chicken, the whole thing is infused in a deeper way than a traditional roast. This is a standard in our house! Just make sure your kitchen shears are sharp and get to spatchcocking, my friend.

Place the chicken on a clean work surface, breast-side down and with the tail end facing you. Using sharp kitchen shears, cut along one side of the backbone. Turn the chicken around and cut along the other side of the backbone and pull it out. Flip over the chicken and firmly press down on the breastbone to flatten the chicken. Dry the skin thoroughly with paper towels. If possible, do this the day before and place in the refrigerator uncovered overnight, allowing the skin to dry out.

Preheat the oven to 425°F.

Arrange the lemon slices in a single layer in the middle of a sheet pan. Top with the garlic cloves and herbs. Place the chicken, skin-side up, on top of the lemon slices.

Using clean hands, rub the softened butter all over the chicken and under the skin of the breasts. Wash your hands and generously sprinkle salt and pepper over the butter and on the underside of the chicken.

Drying the skin of the chicken in the refrigerator overnight allows it to crisp up in the oven.

Add the potatoes to the sheet pan on either side of the chicken. Top the potatoes with the olive oil, mustard, cumin, and salt and pepper to taste. Using clean hands, gently toss the potatoes to coat.

Roast the chicken until a thermometer inserted into the thickest part of the breast reaches 165°F, 45 to 55 minutes. Shake the pan halfway through cooking to ensure that the potatoes don't burn. Remove from the oven and let rest 10 minutes. Transfer the chicken to a cutting board (discard the lemon, garlic, and herbs but keep the pan juices).

Cut the chicken into pieces. Serve with the potatoes and drizzle with the pan juices, which are now infused with incredible flavor from the lemon and herbs.

Variations

Swap the butter for extra-virgin olive oil.

Brussels sprouts are a good alternative to potatoes because they can withstand the longer cook time, and when they're roasted, they sort of taste like potatoes. Just add to the pan and dress with the oil and mustard as you do the potatoes.

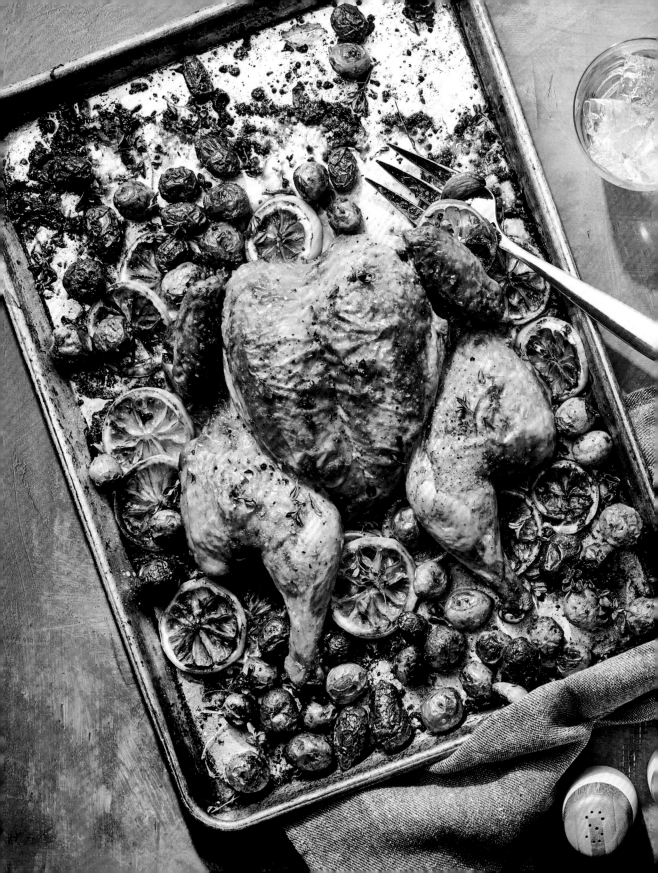

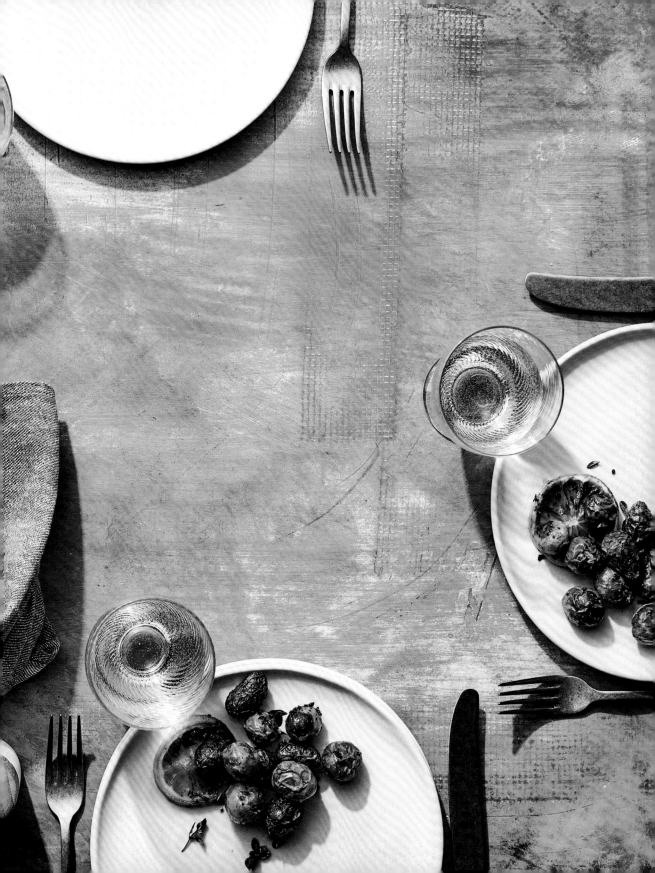

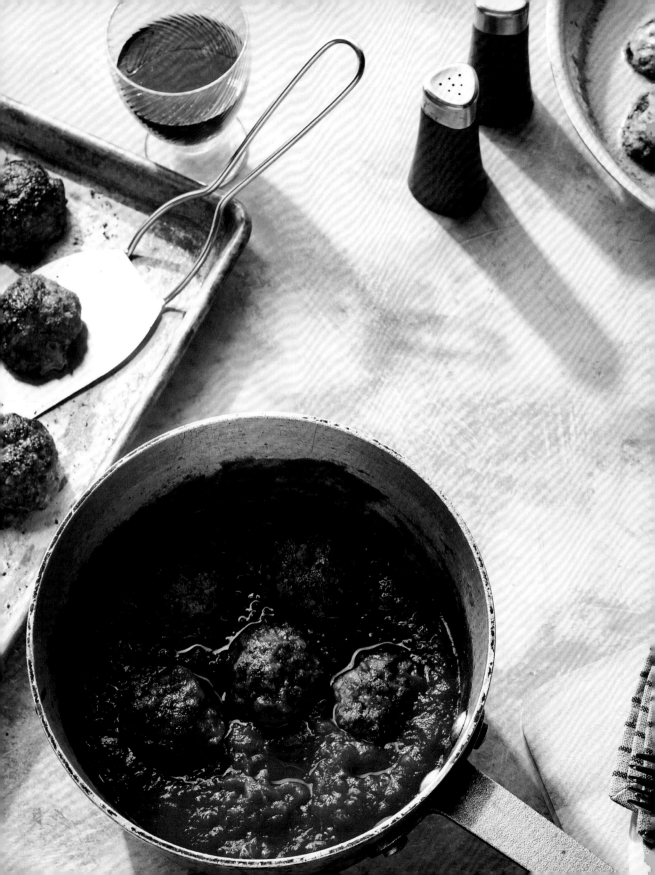

Dinners

Chicken Teriyaki Bowl

SERVES 4
PREP TIME: 15 minutes
TOTAL TIME: 35 minutes

CHICKEN

6 boneless, skinless chicken thighs

1 tablespoon avocado oil
or extra-virgin olive oil

½ teaspoon kosher salt

½ teaspoon freshly ground
black pepper

TERIYAKI SAUCE

1 cup reduced-sodium soy sauce

½ cup honey

1 tablespoon balsamic vinegar

2 teaspoons garlic powder

1 teaspoon ground ginger

1 teaspoon cornstarch

VEGETABLES

2 tablespoons avocado oil
or extra-virgin olive oil

3 cups broccoli florets

3 carrots, peeled and cut into
thin strips

1 cup snap peas or snow peas

FOR SERVING

4 cups cooked rice

Sure, you can buy premade teriyaki sauce, but making it yourself gives you control over the salt and sugar content. As with many of the other recipes, the "bowl" dinner is your starter for great things to come in the future! For a bowl like this, play with the variety of veggies and remember that your kitchen is a laboratory, so have fun experimenting.

Preheat the oven to 425°F.

PREPARE THE CHICKEN: Arrange the chicken thighs on a sheet pan. Drizzle with the oil and sprinkle with the salt and pepper. Roast for 20 to 25 minutes. Flip halfway through.

MAKE THE TERIYAKI SAUCE: In a medium saucepan set over medium heat, whisk together the soy sauce, honey, vinegar, garlic powder, and ginger until fully combined. Reduce the heat and simmer until slightly reduced, about 10 minutes. In a small bowl, whisk the cornstarch and 2 tablespoons water. Add to the saucepan and boil until the sauce thickens. Remove from the heat. (You can make this ahead and store airtight in the refrigerator for up to 2 weeks.)

MEANWHILE, COOK THE VEGETABLES: In a large skillet, heat the oil over medium-high heat. When hot, add the broccoli, carrots, and snap peas and sauté until the broccoli and peas turn a bright green, 3 to 5 minutes.

RECIPE CONTINUES

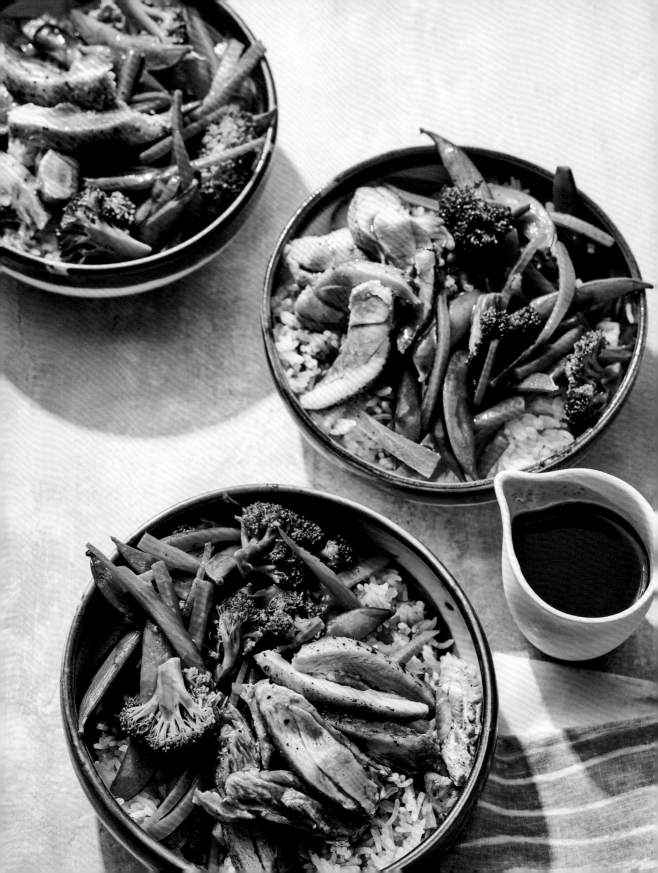

Remove the chicken from the oven, let rest for 5 minutes, then slice into strips.

TO SERVE: Divide the rice among four bowls. Top with the vegetables on one side and the chicken strips on the other side. Drizzle the chicken with room temp or warm teriyaki sauce.

Tia's Tips

I don't cook the chicken *in* the teriyaki sauce for two reasons. First, the sauce burns onto the baking sheet and you lose some of it. Second, you get more teriyaki flavor when you drizzle it over the chicken in the bowl.

Buy cooked rice or make a big batch and freeze half. One less thing to prep!

3-Ingredient Roasted Chicken

SERVES 3 OR 4

PREP TIME: 5 minutes

TOTAL TIME: 1 hour 15 minutes

1 whole chicken (3 to 5 pounds)

Kosher salt and freshly ground black pepper

Tia's Tip

If you have the time, let the chicken sit uncovered in the refrigerator overnight (this dries the skin and makes it crisp up better).

In the last chapter I taught you how to spatchcock a chicken for when you don't have time to roast the whole bird. However, if you have free time, make this on a Sunday and use it for other dishes in this cookbook. Also, it's easy to roast two birds at once, so if you have a lot of humans running around your house, just throw a second one in at the same time.

Preheat the oven to 500°F.

Remove the chicken from the package, remove the giblet bag or neck from the inside cavity (or better yet, ask your butcher to do it for you!). Place the chicken breast-side up on a sheet pan or roasting pan. Pat the chicken dry with a paper towel.

Generously sprinkle salt and pepper all over the chicken, including inside the cavity. Roast until the chicken begins to brown, about 15 minutes. Reduce the oven temperature to 350°F and continue roasting until a thermometer inserted in the thickest part of the breast reaches 165°F, 40 to 50 minutes. If the chicken is browning too quickly, lightly cover with foil.

Remove the chicken to a cutting board and let rest 10 to 15 minutes before carving.

Pork
Lo Mein

SERVES 6

PREP TIME: 15 minutes

TOTAL TIME: 30 minutes

1 pound spaghetti

3 tablespoons neutral oil (such as grapeseed) or cold-pressed sesame oil

2 boneless pork chops (total 8 ounces), cut into ½-inch cubes

Kosher salt and freshly ground black pepper

3 scallions, chopped

3 garlic cloves, minced

1 (12-ounce) bag coleslaw mix or 1½ cups thinly sliced cabbage

8 ounces snow peas

3 tablespoons oyster sauce or fish sauce

3 tablespoons soy sauce

1 tablespoon toasted sesame oil

Sesame seeds (optional)

I adore this quick dish with all of my heart and taste buds; it's faster than piling into the car and picking up takeout, and it's incredibly versatile. Swap the snow peas and pork for other veggie-protein combinations, and you'll never see the end of your options.

Cook the pasta according to the package directions. Drain in a colander and rinse with cold water to stop the pasta from overcooking. Leave in the colander until ready to use.

In a large skillet, heat 2 tablespoons of the neutral oil over medium-high heat. Add the pork and sauté until no longer pink, 3 to 4 minutes. Remove to a plate and sprinkle with a pinch each of salt and pepper.

Add the remaining 1 tablespoon neutral oil to the pan, stir in the scallions, garlic, cabbage slaw, and snow peas and sauté until the cabbage starts to wilt and the snow peas turn a bright green, about 4 minutes.

Toss in the pasta and cooked pork and use tongs to mix the pasta with the veggies. Add the oyster sauce, soy sauce, and toasted sesame oil. Mix to coat all the pasta. Sprinkle with sesame seeds (if using) and salt and pepper to taste and toss again. Serve immediately.

Tia's Tips

Substitute 1 pound cooked shrimp or 2 cups 3-Ingredient Roasted Chicken (page 207) for the pork. Since you don't need to cook them, just add when you toss in the pasta.

Pay attention when purchasing your sesame oil: Cold-pressed sesame oil will be both light in color and flavor, while toasted has a nutty flavor that makes this dish sing!

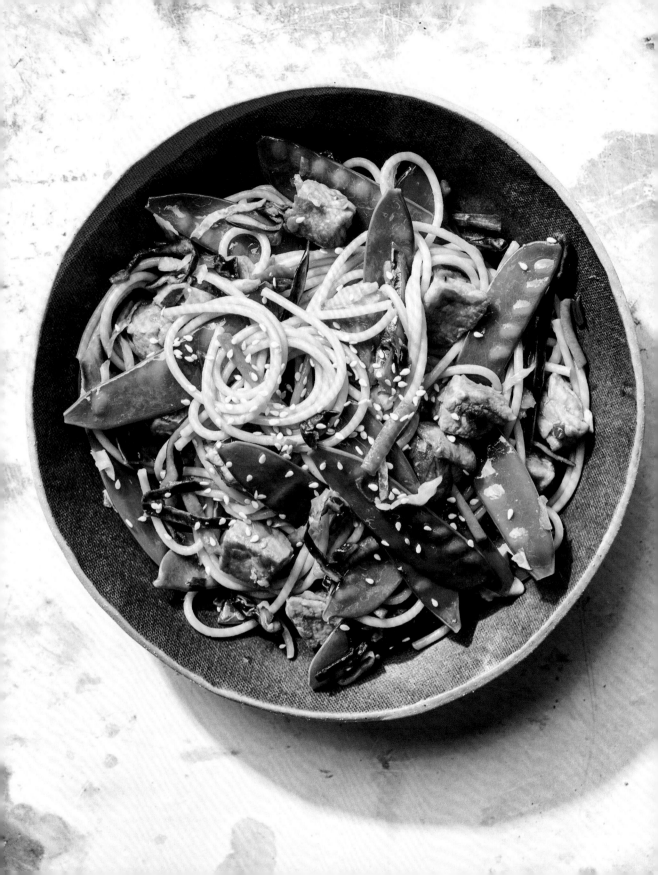

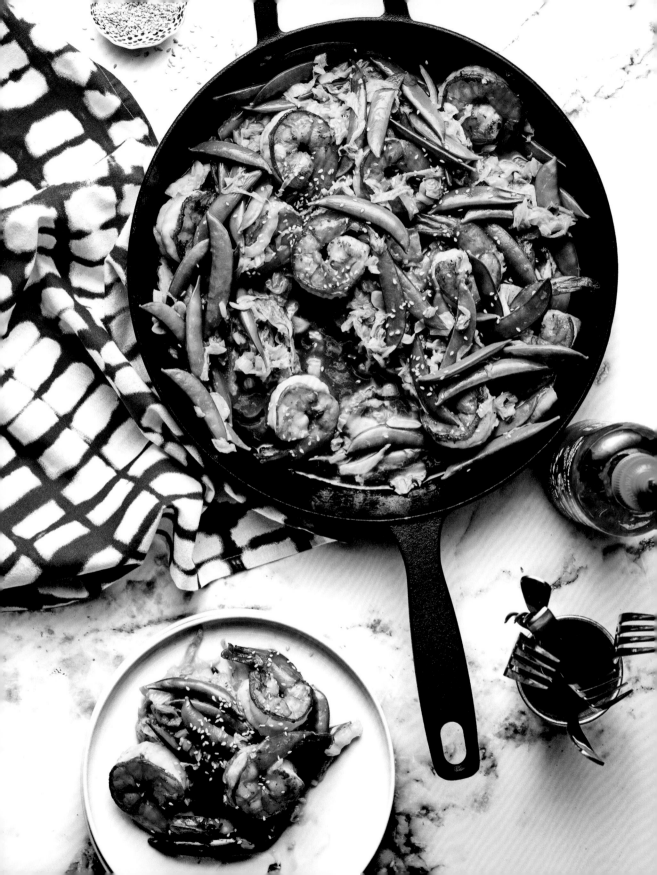

Shrimp Stir-Fry
with Cabbage, Scallions & Snap Peas

SERVES 4 OR 5
PREP TIME: 15 minutes
TOTAL TIME: 25 minutes

3 tablespoons neutral oil

1 bunch scallions, thinly sliced

4 garlic cloves, sliced

4 cups thinly sliced green or
    napa cabbage

3 cups snap peas

⅔ cup chicken or vegetable broth

2 tablespoons reduced-sodium
    soy sauce

2 tablespoons toasted sesame oil

1 teaspoon granulated sugar

2 teaspoons cornstarch

1 pound peeled cooked
    large shrimp

4 cups cooked brown rice or
    cauliflower rice, for serving

1 tablespoon toasted
    sesame seeds,
    for garnish (optional)

Sriracha or chili-garlic sauce,
    for serving (optional)

Stir-fries are the real deal quick fixes. Once you get the technique down, they're versatile and can be easily adapted to the palates of your family as well as to whatever is available in your fridge.

In a large heavy skillet or wok, heat the neutral oil over medium-high heat. Toss in the scallions, garlic, cabbage, and snap peas. Stir occasionally until the cabbage has wilted, about 6 minutes.

Pour the chicken broth into a glass measuring cup. Whisk in the soy sauce, sesame oil, and sugar until combined. Pour into the skillet and toss with the vegetables. In the same measuring cup, whisk the cornstarch and ¼ cup water. Push all the vegetables to the side of the pan and add the cornstarch mixture. Whisk and allow the liquid in the pan to come to a simmer and thicken. Toss in the shrimp and stir until heated.

Serve over rice. If desired, sprinkle with sesame seeds. If you need some heat, add sriracha or chili-garlic sauce.

Tia's Tip

Substitute 2 cups 3-Ingredient Roasted Chicken (page 207) for the shrimp.

Creamy "Alfredo" Pasta

SERVES 4 OR 5

PREP TIME: 15 minutes

TOTAL TIME: 30 minutes

1 pound pasta, such as fettuccine, penne, or fusilli

1 (15-ounce) can white beans or cannellini

2 tablespoons extra-virgin olive oil

4 garlic cloves, grated or minced

5 ounces spinach or kale, chopped

¼ cup grated parmesan cheese or nutritional yeast

1 teaspoon kosher salt

½ teaspoon freshly ground black pepper

This dish has everything: protein, carbs, greens, and flavooorrrr! Growing up, I loved Alfredo for the rich blanket of cream and cheese glazed over every noodle. In adulthood, however, it just makes me feel weighed down. Here's my healthy version that doesn't compromise the heartiness of delectable Alfredo.

Cook the pasta according to the package directions. Reserve about 1 cup of the cooking liquid before draining the pasta.

Meanwhile, drain most of the liquid from the beans. Add the beans along with the remaining liquid to a blender or food processor and blend until smooth.

In a large skillet, heat the oil over medium heat. Add the garlic and sauté just until fragrant, about 30 seconds. Add the pureed beans and ½ cup of the reserved pasta cooking water and mix until combined. Toss in the spinach and stir to wilt.

Add the cooked pasta and toss to cover in the sauce. Stir in another ¼ cup pasta cooking water. If the pasta looks dry, add a bit more pasta water. Sprinkle with the parmesan and toss. Season with the salt and pepper. Serve.

Tia's Tips

Blend the beans until just smooth. Overblending may release too much starch, which will impact the creaminess.

Add some diced chicken for more protein, and switch up the spinach or kale with broccoli and zucchini if you prefer!

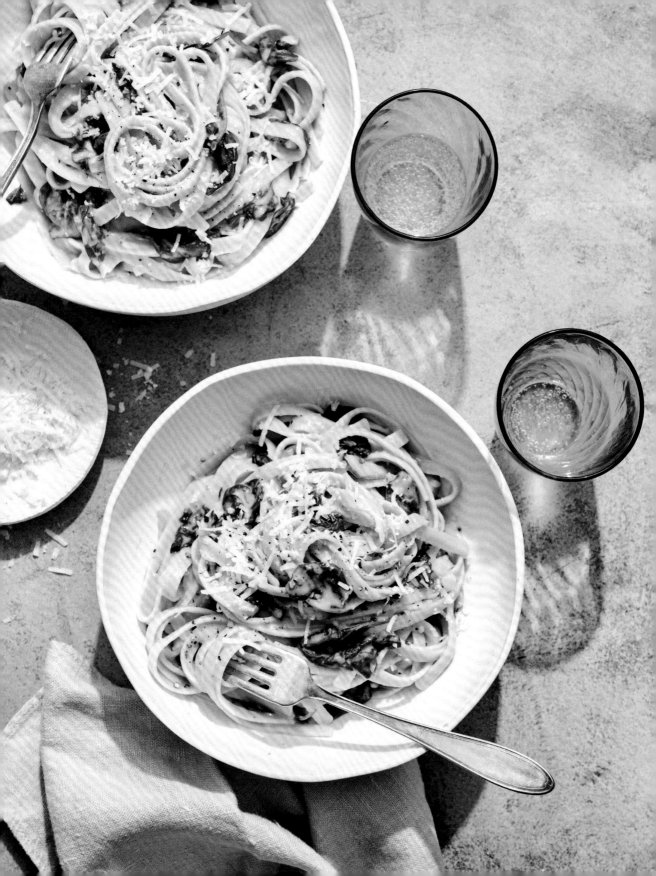

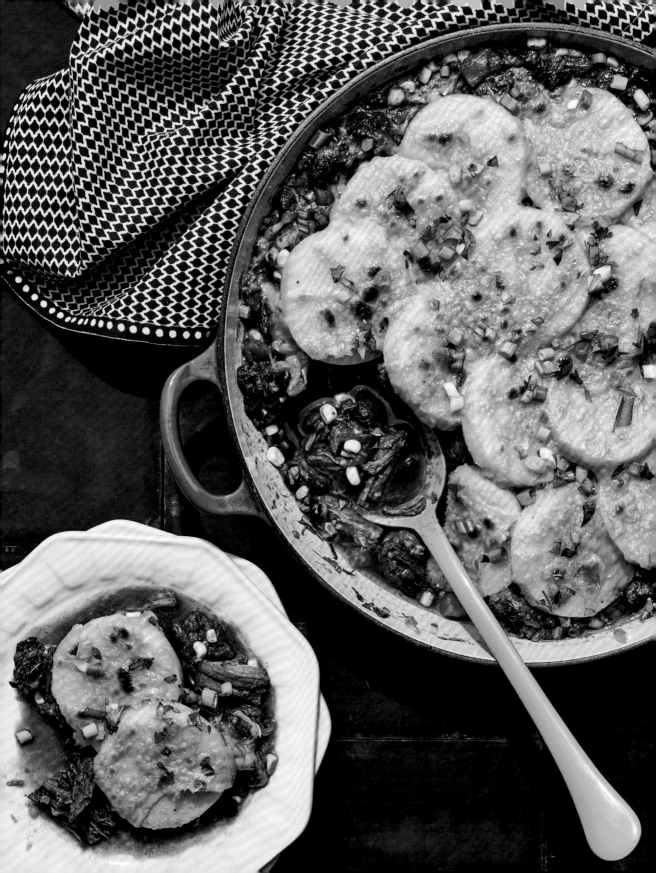

Tex-Mex Shepherd's Pie

SERVES 8 TO 10

PREP TIME: 25 minutes

TOTAL TIME: 3 hours 30 minutes

3 pounds boneless chuck roast, cut into 2- to 3-inch pieces, excess fat trimmed

Spice Rub (page 191)

Extra-virgin olive oil

1 large yellow onion, roughly chopped

2 medium carrots, roughly chopped

2 large cloves garlic, slightly smashed

3 cups beef broth

1 (14.5-ounce) can diced tomatoes

8 sprigs cilantro

1 (4-ounce) can mild diced green chilies

1 tablespoon Worcestershire sauce

2 cups frozen corn kernels

1 (15-ounce) can white beans, rinsed and drained

1 (15-ounce) can black beans, rinsed and drained

2 (1-pound) tubes premade polenta

2 to 3 cups shredded sharp cheddar cheese

GARNISH

Chopped scallions

Chopped cilantro

A twist on a shepherd's pie with amazing Tex-Mex flavors. I use premade polenta as a topping in lieu of the traditional mashed potatoes because it saves on prep time and cleanup. For the meat, I prefer chuck roast, a typically inexpensive cut of beef with beautiful marbleization that encourages the meat to fall apart when cooking low and slow. Okay, okay. Yes, I said "slow." But the time you'll be working on this recipe is quick without a lot of fuss. Once it's on the stove, you just let it do its thing while you kick up your feet.

Season the beef cubes with the spice rub. In a large Dutch oven or large heavy-bottomed pan, heat 2 tablespoons oil over medium-high heat. When hot, add about one-quarter of the beef and sear, flipping so all sides are browned. You want to cook the beef in batches to avoid overcrowding, which will steam the beef rather than brown it. Add more oil as needed for each batch. Remove the beef to a bowl.

Reduce the heat to medium and add the onion, carrots, and garlic. Sauté until the carrots are softened, 5 to 7 minutes. Add 1 cup of the beef broth and use a wooden spoon to scrape up any browned bits on the bottom of the pan. All of these bits (called *fond* in the culinary world) contain incredible flavor, and you don't want to lose them. Stir in the remaining 2 cups beef broth, the canned tomatoes, cilantro, green chilies, beef cubes, and Worcestershire sauce. Cover and bring to a boil, then reduce the heat to low and let

RECIPE CONTINUES

simmer until the beef is tender and easy to shred with a fork, about 2 hours 30 minutes. Remove the beef from the pot to a cutting board and shred with two forks.

Scoop out 1 cup of the cooking liquid from the pot, trying not to get any vegetables in the liquid and discard. Using an immersion blender, blend the remaining cooking liquid and vegetables until slightly chunky. This will help thicken the broth and make it taste creamier. Add the corn and both beans, and return the shredded beef to the stew. Stir until combined.

Slice the polenta into ½-inch-thick rounds. Place the rounds over the stew, overlapping them, and sprinkle with the cheddar. Over medium heat, place the lid back on the pot and allow the polenta to warm up and the cheese to melt, about 5 minutes. (Alternatively, place under the broiler for a few minutes.)

To serve, scoop out a polenta round plus the filling underneath it and place in a bowl. Garnish with scallions and cilantro.

Tia's Tips

You can cook this in a slow cooker, too. Just sear the beef first, then add to the inner pot of a slow cooker with the remaining ingredients. Cook on low for 10 to 12 hours. Follow the directions above after the beef is cooked.

Use any leftover shredded beef in quesadillas and pastas, or make a gravy and serve with mashed potatoes, or use on a loaded potato (see page 223).

Who Doesn't Love Meatballs?

**MAKES 30 MINI OR
15 LARGE MEATBALLS**

PREP TIME: 15 minutes

TOTAL TIME: 33 minutes

½ cup panko bread crumbs

½ cup whole milk

1 large egg

¼ cup grated parmesan cheese

1 tablespoon chopped
 fresh parsley

1 teaspoon kosher salt

1 teaspoon garlic powder

1 teaspoon onion powder

½ teaspoon freshly ground
 black pepper

1 pound ground beef or turkey

Extra-virgin olive oil

Quick Tomato Sauce or
 Creamy "Swedish" Sauce
 (recipes follow)

½ cup shredded
 mozzarella cheese (optional)

⅓ cup sour cream (optional)

Cooked pasta, rice, polenta,
 or grits, for serving

The best dish ever created is meatballs. Okay, maybe not *ever*, but it's up there. You can serve them so many different ways, with a variety of flavors and sauces (I've given you two options here), as an entrée, in soups, for appetizers, and as a snack, too!

Preheat the oven to 400°F.

In a large bowl, mix the panko, milk, egg, parmesan, parsley, salt, garlic powder, onion powder, and pepper until fully combined. Add the meat and gently mix. You don't want to overmix as it tends to make the meatballs dry. This mixture is wet, so the mix will be a little sticky, but that gives the meatballs wonderful moisture inside. Divide the meat mixture into 15 or 30 portions and gently roll into 15 largeish meatballs or 30 mini meatballs. Place on a baking sheet until all the meat has been rolled.

In a large skillet, heat enough oil to cover the bottom of the pan over medium-high heat until hot. Working in batches, add a few meatballs at a time and brown the outsides of the balls. Don't worry if the inside is not cooked because it will finish in the oven. Add more oil to the pan as needed for each batch.

IF SERVING WITH QUICK TOMATO SAUCE: Return the meatballs to the baking sheet and transfer to the oven. Bake until cooked through, 10 minutes for mini meatballs and 15 to 18 minutes for larger meatballs. Make the tomato sauce in a broilerproof skillet and when the meatballs are baked, place them in the skillet and top with the mozzarella (if using).

RECIPE CONTINUES

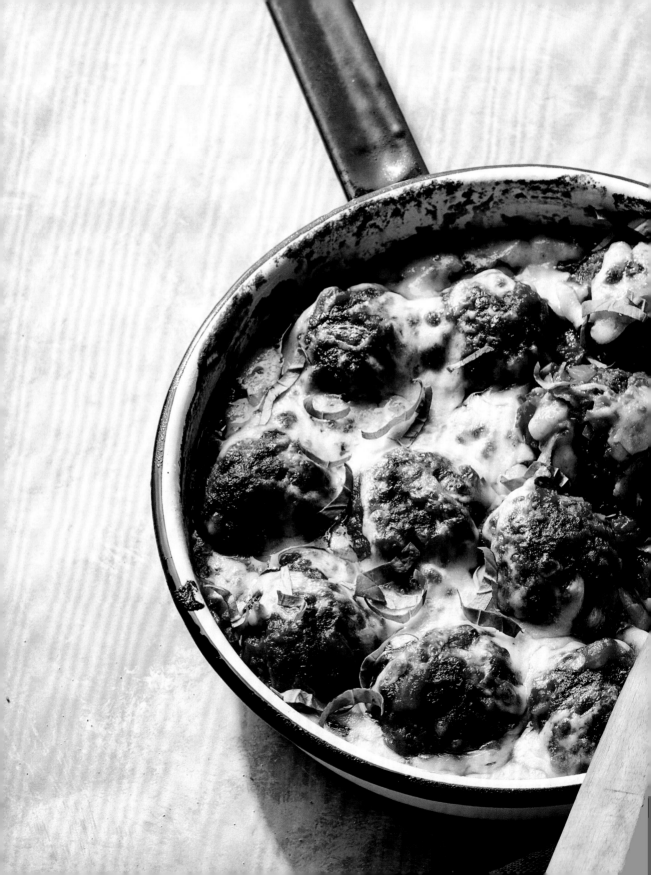

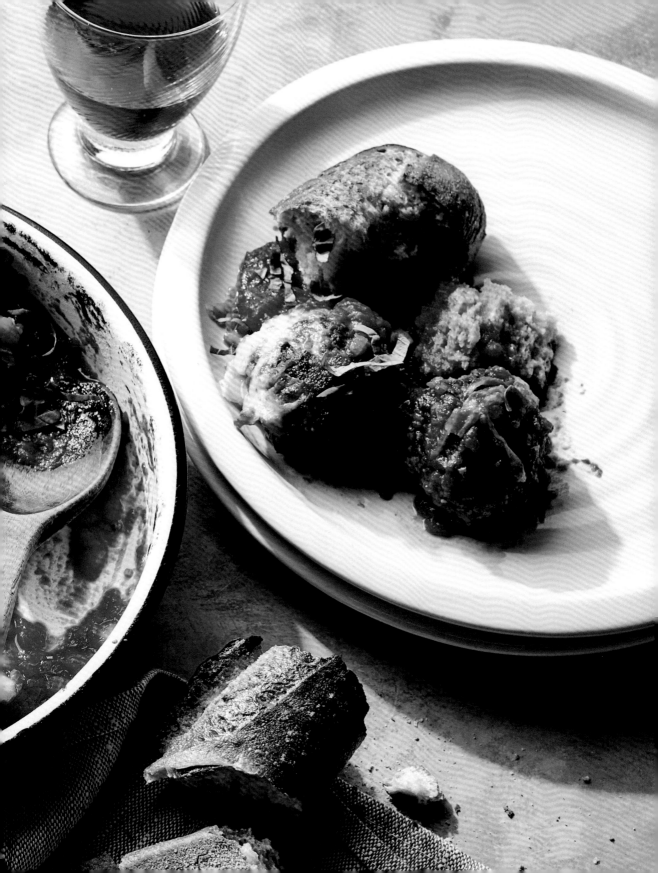

Place under the broiler to melt the cheese. Serve with pasta, rice, or polenta.

IF SERVING WITH THE CREAMY "SWEDISH" SAUCE: Make the sauce as directed. Add the browned meatballs to the sauce and simmer for 5 minutes for mini meatballs and 10 to 15 minutes for larger meatballs. Remove the meatballs to a plate. Stir in the sour cream (if using) and allow the sauce to thicken for 5 minutes. Return the meatballs to the sauce and serve over pasta, rice, or grits.

QUICK TOMATO SAUCE

MAKES 3½ CUPS
PREP TIME: 5 MINUTES
TOTAL TIME: 30 MINUTES

¼ cup extra-virgin olive oil

1 small onion, grated

3 garlic cloves, grated

1 (28-ounce) can
    crushed tomatoes

2 tablespoons tomato paste

1 teaspoon kosher salt

1 teaspoon freshly ground
    black pepper

Use this sauce for pasta or pizza as well as for cooking meatballs. It is a quick tomato sauce that doesn't have any sugar, like some of the jarred sauces.

In a deep skillet, heat the oil over medium-high heat. When the oil is hot, add the onion and sauté for 5 minutes, or until soft. Add garlic and sauté for another minute. Add the canned tomatoes, tomato paste, salt, and pepper and stir well. Let simmer for 20 minutes, stirring occasionally so it doesn't stick to the pan.

CREAMY "SWEDISH" SAUCE

MAKES 4 CUPS

PREP TIME: 5 MINUTES

TOTAL TIME: 30 MINUTES

5 tablespoons unsalted butter

½ small onion, grated

3 cups beef broth

½ cup whole milk or half-and-half

1 tablespoon Worcestershire
    sauce

1 teaspoon Dijon mustard

1 teaspoon kosher salt

¾ teaspoon freshly ground
    black pepper

In a deep skillet, melt the butter over medium heat. Add the onion and sauté until soft, 3 to 5 minutes. Stir in the beef broth, milk, Worcestershire sauce, mustard, salt, and pepper. Bring to a boil over medium high heat. Allow to boil for a few minutes, then reduce the heat to low. Keep warm until ready to use.

Tia's Tips

Meatballs freeze so well; you can double the recipe or even triple it.

Kids love rolling meatballs into ball shapes, but be careful of the raw meat. Have them wear gloves or make sure they wash their hands really well (one full birthday song!).

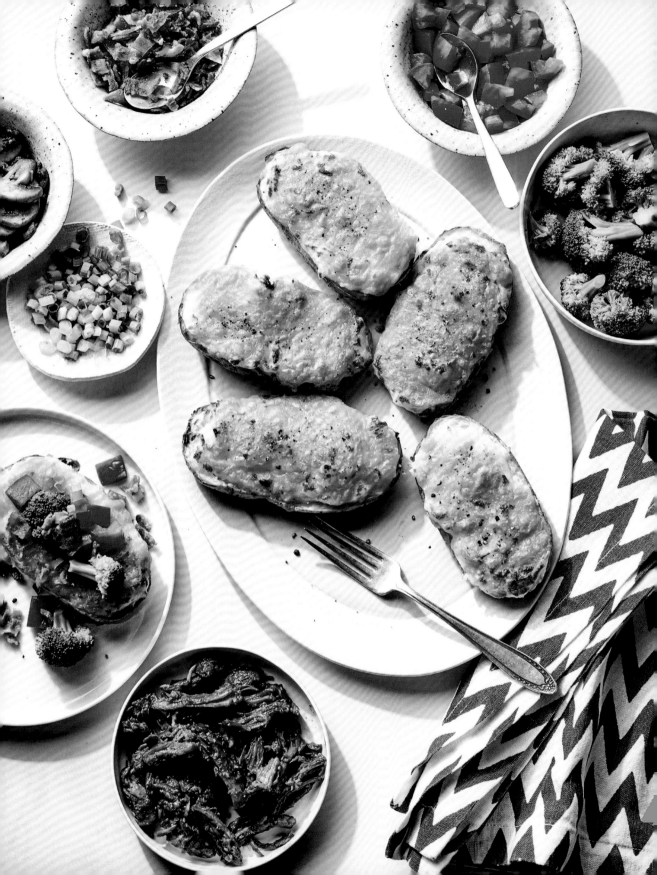

Loaded Potato Bar

SERVES 4

PREP TIME: 5 minutes

TOTAL TIME: 1 hour

4 medium-to-large russet
potatoes, well scrubbed

1 tablespoon extra-virgin olive oil

⅔ cup whole milk, warmed

4 tablespoons (½ stick)
unsalted butter

Kosher salt and freshly ground
black pepper

TOPPINGS

Cooked broccoli

Chopped cooked bacon

Shredded cheese

Chili

Salsa

Guacamole

Pulled pork or beef

Cooked ground turkey

Sour cream or Greek yogurt

Sautéed mushrooms

Cream of spinach

Tia's Tips

You can use sweet potatoes,
too, for this recipe.

Double the recipe so you can
have potatoes anytime.

Baked potatoes—what a classic! I love that you can customize them however you like, and that every bite is a memory from the past. I also love that they can be sides or meals in themselves.

Preheat the oven to 450°F. Line a large baking sheet with foil.

Using a dinner fork or a small paring knife, poke the potatoes at least 10 times on all sides. Place the potatoes on the lined baking sheet.

Drizzle the potatoes with the oil and use clean hands to rub the oil all over. Bake until you can easily pierce with a knife, 50 to 60 minutes. Remove from the oven and let sit until cool enough to handle; be careful, they will be *hot*.

Place on a cutting board and halve each potato lengthwise. Using a spoon, scoop out the potato flesh into a large bowl, keeping about ¼ inch of the flesh attached to the skin. Don't worry if you punctured a hole in the skin. Place the scooped potatoes cut-side up on the baking sheet.

To the large bowl with the potato flesh, add the warm milk, butter, 2 teaspoons salt, and 1 teaspoon pepper. Mash until fully combined and taste for seasoning. Spoon the potato mixture back into the potato skins. To keep warm, turn the oven down to 200°F and place into the oven. (The potatoes can be made ahead to this point the day before; cover and refrigerate. Or you can freeze them for later.)

Serve warm as a potato bar and have everyone put on their favorite toppings. If cheese is one of the toppings you choose, place under the broiler for a few minutes to melt it.

Pan-Seared Garlic Herb Steak
with Creamy Chimichurri

SERVES 4 OR 5

PREP TIME: 25 minutes

TOTAL TIME: 45 minutes

CREAMY CHIMICHURRI

2 cups firmly packed
parsley leaves

2 cups firmly packed
cilantro leaves

3 or 4 garlic cloves, grated

1 bunch scallions,
coarsely chopped

2 tablespoons sherry vinegar
or juice of 2 limes

1 teaspoon kosher salt

⅛ teaspoon freshly ground
black pepper

⅓ cup extra-virgin olive oil,
plus more as needed

1 large or 2 small avocados,
halved and pitted

STEAK

2 New York strip steaks
(8 ounces each),
about 1½ inches thick

1 teaspoon kosher salt

1 teaspoon freshly ground
black pepper

1 tablespoon olive oil

2 tablespoons unsalted butter

5 garlic cloves, peeled and
slightly smashed

2 or 3 sprigs rosemary or thyme

You'll want to use this creamy chimichurri for everything: fish, chicken, dipping chips, dipping your spoon or finger. Everything. It's as refreshing as the first day of spring, and it will be on repeat.

MAKE THE CREAMY CHIMICHURRI: In a blender or food processor, combine the parsley, cilantro, garlic, scallions, vinegar, salt, and pepper. Pulse several times until all the ingredients are chopped. Add the oil and blend until smooth. Scoop in the avocado flesh and blend until the avocado has pureed into sauce. Serve immediately or refrigerate. If chilled, return to room temperature before serving. This sauce keeps for a week or two in an airtight container.

COOK THE STEAK: Bring the steaks to room temperature for 30 minutes; this helps cook the steak evenly and quicker.

Right before cooking, season the steaks on both sides with the salt and pepper. Heat a cast-iron skillet over high heat until white wisps of smoke appear. Add the olive oil and swirl in the pan. Add the steaks and do not touch them. You want to create a crust on the meat. Cook for 3 to 5 minutes on one side. Flip and cook for another 3 minutes.

Reduce the heat to medium-low and add the butter, garlic, and rosemary to the pan. Carefully tilt the pan toward you so the butter slides to one side. Cook for another 2 minutes, basting the steaks with butter constantly. Remove the steaks

RECIPE CONTINUES

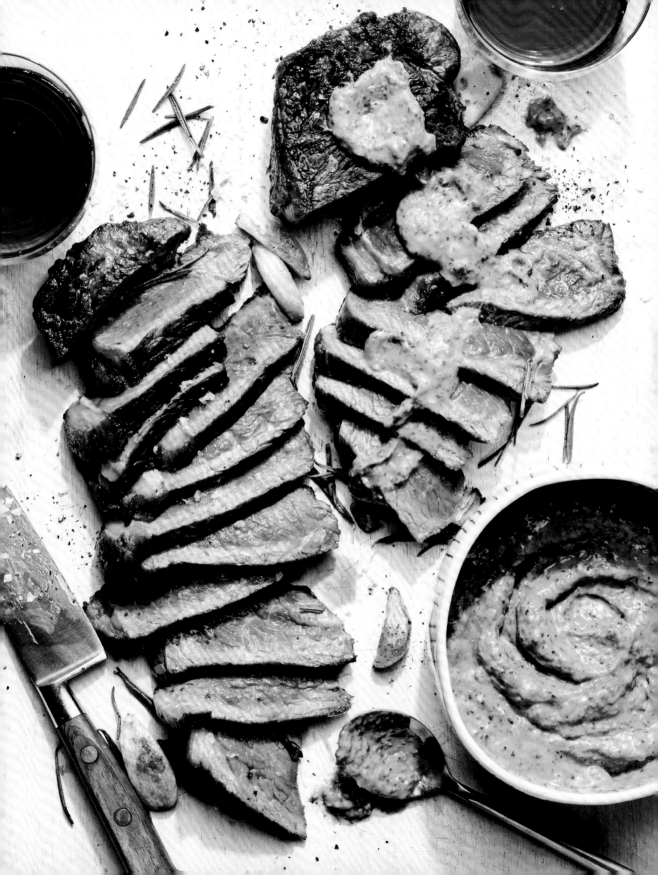

from the pan to a cutting board. Loosely cover with foil and let rest for 10 minutes. This cooking method gives you a medium-rare to medium steak. If you want your steak well done, place in a preheated 400°F oven for 5 to 7 minutes.

Slice the steak across the grain and on a diagonal to the cutting board. Serve with the creamy chimichurri sauce.

Tia's Tips

If you're short on parsley, you can add up to 1 cup of another leafy soft herb, such as mint or basil (not rosemary or thyme). This is a great job for little ones—have them pull the herb leaves off the stems.

This method works well with rib-eye steak and filet mignon. Cooking times may change a bit; just look for the outside to brown and when you poke the middle of the steak with a clean finger, you want it to bounce back.

Super Nachos
with Vegan Cheese Sauce

SERVES 4 TO 6

PREP TIME: 25 minutes

TOTAL TIME: 25 minutes

VEGAN CHEESE SAUCE

2 tablespoons extra-virgin olive oil

1 medium yellow onion, coarsely chopped

2 cups cauliflower florets

3 carrots, sliced into thin rounds

3 garlic cloves, chopped

1½ cups vegetable broth, plus more as needed

2 tablespoons reduced-sodium soy sauce

½ cup raw cashews

2 tablespoons nutritional yeast

1 teaspoon kosher salt

NACHOS

1 tablespoon olive oil

1 pound ground turkey

2 tablespoons Spice Rub (page 191) or 1 (1-ounce) packet taco seasoning

1 (16-ounce) bag corn tortilla chips

You read that right! Vegan cheese! If you're not familiar with nutritional yeast, it has cheesy, nutty, and savory notes used in vegan cooking to emulate the flavor of cheese. For this recipe, you may wonder, "Wait, is this Velveeta?" But no, it most certainly isn't. Get this: They call the yeast "nutritional" because it contains protein, vitamins, minerals, and antioxidants.

MAKE THE VEGAN CHEESE SAUCE: In a saucepan, heat the oil over medium heat. When hot, add the onion, cauliflower, carrots, and garlic and sauté until the onions are soft, 3 to 5 minutes. Add the vegetable broth, soy sauce, and cashews and bring to a simmer. Cover the pan and let cook until the cauliflower and carrots are easily pierced with a fork, about 5 minutes. Uncover and let cool slightly.

Add the slightly cooled vegetable mixture to a blender with the salt and nutritional yeast. Remove the steam vent from the center of the blender lid and hold a kitchen towel over the hole. Carefully puree until smooth, adding more vegetable broth if needed for texture.

PREPARE THE NACHOS: In a large skillet, heat the oil over medium-high heat. Add the turkey and use a wooden spoon to break up any large chunks (you want crumbly meat) and brown until the turkey is no longer pink, about 7 minutes. Sprinkle the spice rub over the meat and toss until the meat is covered in spices. Keep warm until ready to assemble.

RECIPE + INGREDIENTS CONTINUE

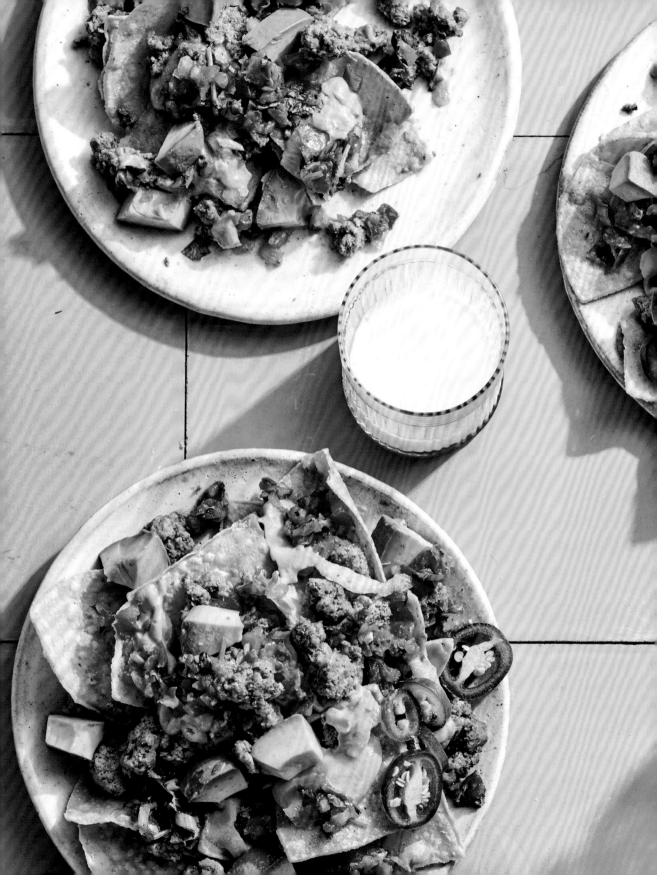

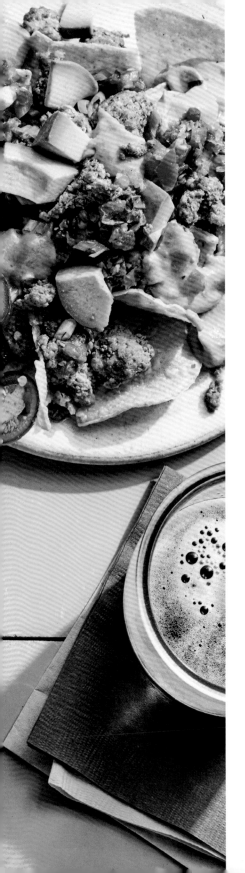

TOPPINGS

Chopped tomatoes

Salsa

Chopped cilantro

Guacamole

Avocado cubes

Sliced jalapeños

Chopped scallions

On individual plates, lay a handful of chips and top with the cooked turkey. Drizzle the cheese sauce over the turkey and chips. Serve with bowls of your family's favorite toppings.

Tia's Tips

This cheese sauce is very versatile. You can dip bread and chips into it or pour it over cooked vegetables and pasta. You can even eat it as a soup with broccoli.

Remember to be careful when adding hot liquid to a blender. The steam vent should be removed from the lid (or if there is no steam vent, the lid should be off-center) and a kitchen towel should be placed on top of the lid to stop the liquid from volcano-ing out. Also, most important, fill only half full at a time.

This sauce is easy to freeze. Make extra and portion it for easy weeknight dinners.

You can be quick about chopping the vegetables for the sauce. Just give them a rough chop since they get blended anyway.

Ground turkey can be swapped out for beef, beans, or lentils. Cook the same way as you would the turkey.

Meatloaf Cupcakes
with Mashed Potato Frosting

SERVES 4
PREP TIME: 15 minutes
TOTAL TIME: 40 minutes

MEATLOAF CUPCAKES

Nonstick cooking spray

1 pound ground beef or turkey (85% lean)

1 large egg

1 medium onion, grated

¼ cup fine, dried bread crumbs

¼ cup whole milk

¼ cup ketchup

2 tablespoons soy sauce or Worcestershire sauce

2 tablespoons chopped fresh parsley

1 teaspoon garlic powder

1 teaspoon kosher salt

1 teaspoon freshly ground black pepper

MASHED POTATO FROSTING

4 medium-to-large russet potatoes, peeled and cut into large chunks

⅔ cup whole milk, warmed

4 tablespoons (½ stick) unsalted butter

2 teaspoons kosher salt

1 teaspoon freshly ground black pepper

Chopped parsley, for garnish

Meatloaf needs a little rebranding, don't you think? Like, served in cupcake form? Yep! Rather than plopping a loaf onto the table, serve up cute little servings in the shape of everyone's favorite dessert!

Preheat the oven to 375°F. Lightly spritz 8 cups of a muffin tin with cooking spray or line with paper liners.

MAKE THE MEATLOAF CUPCAKES: In a large bowl, combine the beef, egg, onion, bread crumbs, milk, ketchup, soy sauce, parsley, garlic powder, salt, and pepper. Using clean hands, mix until combined, but do not overmix. Scoop into the prepared muffin cups and gently push down. Bake until the meat is no longer pink, 20 to 25 minutes.

MEANWHILE, MAKE THE MASHED POTATO FROSTING: Fill a large soup pot two-thirds with water. Add the potatoes and bring to a boil over medium high heat. Cook until you can easily pierce all the potatoes with a fork or knife, about 10 minutes. Drain.

Transfer the potatoes to a large bowl and slightly mash. Add the warm milk, butter, salt, and pepper and mash until fully combined.

Remove the meatloaf cupcakes from the oven and place on a platter or serving plate. Using an ice cream scoop, scoop the mashed potatoes on top of the cupcakes. Sprinkle the potatoes with parsley and serve. Store leftovers in airtight containers in the refrigerator.

The mashed potatoes can be made ahead of time. I like to use a potato masher to make mashed potatoes because mixers often overdo it and the potatoes become gummy. Kids can do the mashing, too.

Tia's Tips

A usual serving is 2 sliders for this size, but don't be shocked if the kids ask for a third. If you have any left over, it packs easily for a school lunch.

If you're thinking "I will never use celery salt in any other recipes," think again. Try it on popcorn, potatoes, rice, cooked vegetables or in soups. The combination of salt and celery enhances bland foods in need of not only salt, but subtle, tangy flavor. It also has a two-year shelf life. Long live celery salt!

Grating the onion means it will melt into the sliders while they cook, rather than having a crunchy texture if diced.

Can't Eat Just One Oven Slider

MAKES 4 OR 5 SLIDERS

PREP TIME: 10 minutes

TOTAL TIME: 35 minutes

Nonstick cooking spray

½ small yellow onion

1 pound ground beef (85% lean)

1 large egg

1 tablespoon spicy brown mustard

1 teaspoon Worcestershire sauce

1 teaspoon celery salt

½ teaspoon freshly ground
    black pepper

4 or 5 mini hamburger buns
    or pretzel buns

Sliced cheese

My kids are thrilled anytime I make sliders. Something about the mini burgers really tickles them, and if something as simple as a little burger brings them joy, I'm gonna give it to them! Being the juiciest, most flavorful sliders you will ever have is just the cherry (ahem . . . cheese!) on top.

Preheat the oven to 400°F. Spritz a baking sheet with cooking spray.

Grate the onion on the large holes of a box grater. The onion will be wet, so gently squeeze out some moisture before placing in a large bowl.

Add the ground beef, egg, mustard, Worcestershire sauce, celery salt, and pepper to the bowl with the onion. Gently mix all the ingredients without overmixing. Using a ⅓-cup measuring cup, gently pack the meat mixture and shake to release little discs. Place the formed patties on the prepared baking sheet 2 inches apart. With the bottom of the measuring cup, push down to slightly flatten.

Transfer to the oven and bake for 25 minutes, flipping the sliders after 15 minutes. When the sliders are 5 minutes from being done, place the buns in the oven and top the sliders with cheese.

Remove from the oven and assemble the sliders.

Chicken Satay
with a Creamy Dipping Sauce

**SERVES 4 OR 5 AS AN
ENTRÉE OR 10 TO 12 AS
AN APPETIZER**

PREP TIME: 15 minutes

TOTAL TIME: 4 hours 20 minutes

CHICKEN

⅔ cup full-fat canned
  coconut milk

Juice of 1 lime

3 tablespoons Thai red
  curry paste

2 pounds thin-cut chicken breast
  cutlets or tenders

Nonstick cooking spray (optional)

DIPPING SAUCE

1 cup creamy peanut butter,
  almond butter,
  or sunflower butter

Juice of 1 lime

¼ cup soy sauce

¼ cup water or coconut milk

2 tablespoons light brown sugar

2 teaspoons fish sauce

2 garlic cloves, chopped, or
  ½ teaspoon garlic powder

½ teaspoon ground ginger

½ teaspoon sriracha (optional)

Kosher salt and freshly ground
  black pepper

FOR SERVING

Chopped cilantro

Chopped peanuts (optional)

If Thai red curry paste is new to you, then meet your MVP "time-saver ingredient," which is jam-packed with so much flavor your mouth will be transported to another time and place. Asian sauces often call for a lot of ingredients—fresh herbs, spices, you name it—to achieve the perfect balance of sweet, sour, and spicy. Sometimes, I opt for premade stuff, like the red curry paste in this recipe, to cut back on all those ingredients and all that prep. You'll find it in the Asian section at the market.

MARINATE THE CHICKEN: In a large zip-top bag, combine the coconut milk, lime juice, and red curry paste. Reseal the bag tightly and mix all the ingredients together.

Place the chicken cutlets or tenders on a work surface. Cover with plastic wrap and pound the chicken until ¼ to ½ inch thick. Cut into 1½-inch-wide strips. Add the chicken to the marinade and refrigerate for at least 4 hours or overnight.

MEANWHILE, MAKE THE DIPPING SAUCE: To a blender, add the creamy peanut butter, lime juice, soy sauce, water or coconut milk, light brown sugar, fish sauce, garlic, ground ginger, sriracha (if using), and salt and pepper. Blend until fully combined. If the sauce is too thick, add 1 tablespoon of hot water at a time to loosen. The sauce should be pourable. Serve in a small bowl next to the chicken skewers.

There are two ways to cook this chicken: on a grill pan or in the oven. The grill pan will give it char marks and infuse a light smoky flavor. The oven will let you cook all the chicken

RECIPE CONTINUES

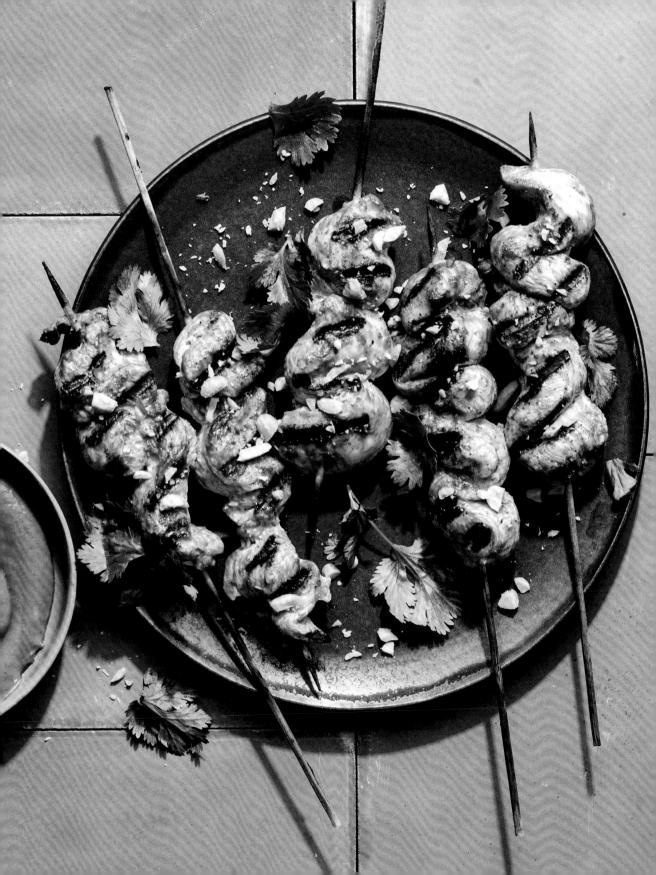

at once. If you will be cooking these under the broiler, soak twenty 10-inch skewers in water for 1 hour to prevent their burning. No need to soak if cooking on a grill pan.

Remove the chicken strips from the marinade and thread onto the skewers so that the strip of chicken will lay flat and not bunch up—this allows the chicken to cook evenly.

Preheat a grill pan over medium-high heat or preheat the broiler.

Spritz the grill pan with cooking spray. Place the chicken skewers on the grill pan. Grill until there is no longer any pink, 2 to 3 minutes per side. Or place the skewers on a sheet pan and broil for 2 to 3 minutes, remove the chicken, and flip to cook the other side for another 1 to 2 minutes, until the juices run clear.

TO SERVE: Garnish the chicken with chopped cilantro and nuts (if using). Serve with the dipping sauce on the side.

Tia's Tips

Nowadays, you can find both thin-cut chicken breast cutlets as well as tenders—big time-savers here. If you can find only whole chicken breasts, you will have to first slice them horizontally in half to get thinner pieces. However, even if you start with cutlets or tenders, you still have to pound them flat (a brilliant stress reliever!), but it's easier than starting with the whole breast.

Marinating in a resealable bag (instead of a baking dish) saves space in my refrigerator, speeds up the process of infusing flavors into the chicken when you remove the air from the bag, and makes for easy cleanup!

This dipping sauce works great as a dressing; just thin it out with a little bit of water if it's too thick (go light, with 1 tablespoon at a time) or toss with some cooked spaghetti and enjoy cold sesame noodles.

If the spice of sriracha is intimidating, start with a smaller amount and add slowly. The sriracha helps balance out the sweet and sour without making it spicy.

Lazy Mom Lasagna

SERVES 4 OR 5

PREP TIME: 10 minutes

TOTAL TIME: 1 hour

1 (25-ounce) jar tomato sauce (or Quick Tomato Sauce on page 220)

1 (25-ounce) bag frozen ravioli

3 cups frozen chopped broccoli florets

1 cup shredded mozzarella cheese

Tia's Tips

Treat this recipe as a rough guideline. Feel free to use more ravioli (any type you want!), veggies, or cheese. I like using frozen broccoli because it is easy and pairs well with the flavors. I also love sautéed spinach, frozen green beans, and mixed vegetables; just make sure they are bite-size.

Double the recipe and use a 9 x 13-inch baking dish to feed a large group. You may even have leftovers!

Normally, lasagna calls for all sorts of mixing bowls, pots, pans, and a flurry of steps. Not here! By using ravioli instead of pasta sheets, you've eliminated boiling and drying the noodles and mixing the cheese. All the work is done for you! Well, except for the layering, but that's simple, especially if you assign someone else to do it.

Preheat the oven to 400°F.

In the bottom of a 9 × 9-inch baking dish, spread 1 cup of the tomato sauce. Make a layer of frozen ravioli (about 16) on top of the sauce. Sprinkle with 1½ cups of the broccoli and ⅓ cup of the mozzarella cheese, then dollop with about ½ cup tomato sauce. Repeat with 16 more ravioli, 1½ cups broccoli, ⅓ cup mozzarella, and ½ cup sauce. Cover with the remaining ravioli, ½ cup tomato sauce, and remaining ⅓ cup mozzarella. Cover the baking dish with foil.

Transfer to the oven and bake until the sauce bubbles up in the pan, 35 to 40 minutes. Remove the foil and bake for another 10 minutes to lightly brown the cheese topping.

Remove from the oven and let sit about 5 to 10 minutes before serving.

Homemade Pizza Bar

MAKES TWO 9-INCH PIZZAS OR ONE 18-INCH PIZZA

PREP TIME: 25 minutes

TOTAL TIME: 1 hour 5 minutes
(includes 15 minutes of resting time)

2 cups all-purpose flour, plus more for kneading the dough

2½ teaspoons baking powder

1 tablespoon grated parmesan cheese (optional)

1 teaspoon kosher salt

½ teaspoon garlic powder (optional)

½ teaspoon onion powder (optional)

¾ cup water

2 tablespoons extra-virgin olive oil, plus more for the pans

TOPPINGS

Marinara sauce

Mozzarella cheese

Pepperoni

Sliced fennel

Crumbled cooked sausage

Caramelized onion

Olives

Fresh mushrooms

Cooked veggies

Enjoy homemade pizza or pizza roll-ups with this simple, no-yeast recipe. Every eater in the household will be satisfied when making their own personal-size pizza, which encourages new, creative topping combos! For a playful school lunch, roll up, bake, and cut into wheels. Easy to pack and fun to eat (even at room temperature!).

In a large bowl, whisk together the flour, baking powder, parmesan (if using), salt, garlic powder (if using), and onion powder (if using). Stir in the water and oil with a silicone spatula, until all the ingredients are combined and a dough forms. Lightly flour a clean work surface and knead the dough for 1 to 2 minutes (don't overknead). Shape into a ball and return to the bowl. Cover with a towel and let sit for 15 minutes while you're getting the toppings ready (you can prepare the dough a couple of hours ahead and leave at room temperature).

Preheat the oven to 400°F. Line a sheet pan (or two if you are making two 9-inch pizzas) with parchment paper or generously grease with extra-virgin olive oil.

If making small pizzas, cut the dough in half. Lightly flour the surface. Gently push the dough with clean fingertips and form into a round disc. Using a rolling pin, roll out to a round ¼ inch thick. Place the rolled dough on the prepared sheet pan. Top with marinara sauce, mozzarella, and any other toppings. Repeat with the second piece of dough.

Tia's Tip

If making individual pizzas, write everyone's name on the parchment paper next to their pizza.

Bake until the dough is golden brown on the underside of the pizza, 15 to 20 minutes, rotating the pizza halfway through cooking.

Remove from the oven. Transfer to a cutting board, slice, and serve.

Variation

PIZZA ROLL-UPS: Divide the pizza dough in half. With a rolling pin, roll one of the pieces of dough to an 11 × 7-inch rectangle. Spread marinara sauce all over, leaving a 1-inch border on all sides. Top with cheese and toppings. Starting with a long side, roll up the dough. Place the roll seam-side down on a prepared baking sheet. Bake at 400°F until the dough is golden brown, 20 to 22 minutes. Remove from the oven and let sit 5 minutes before slicing into 1-inch-wide discs. Serve with more marinara sauce for dipping, if you like.

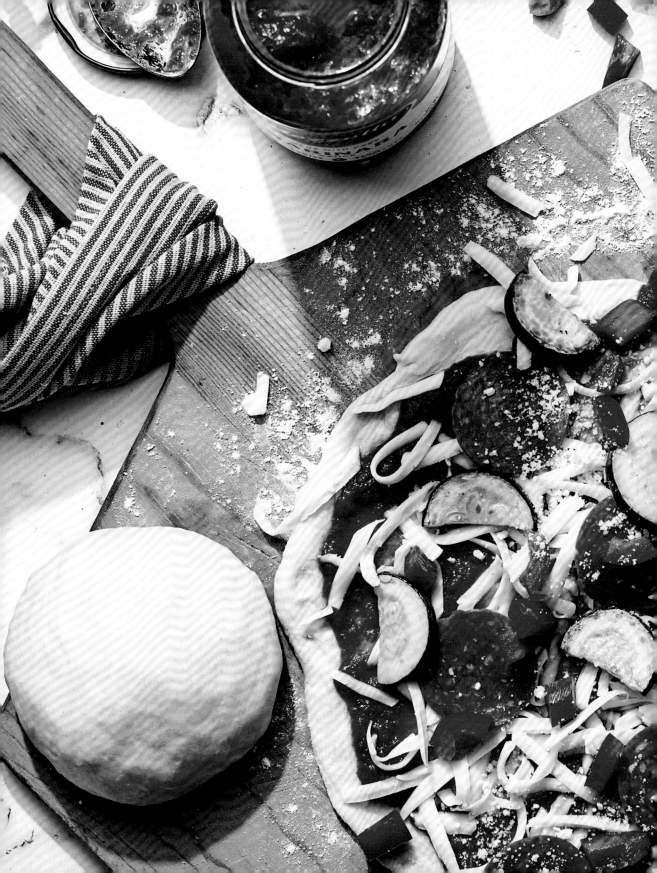

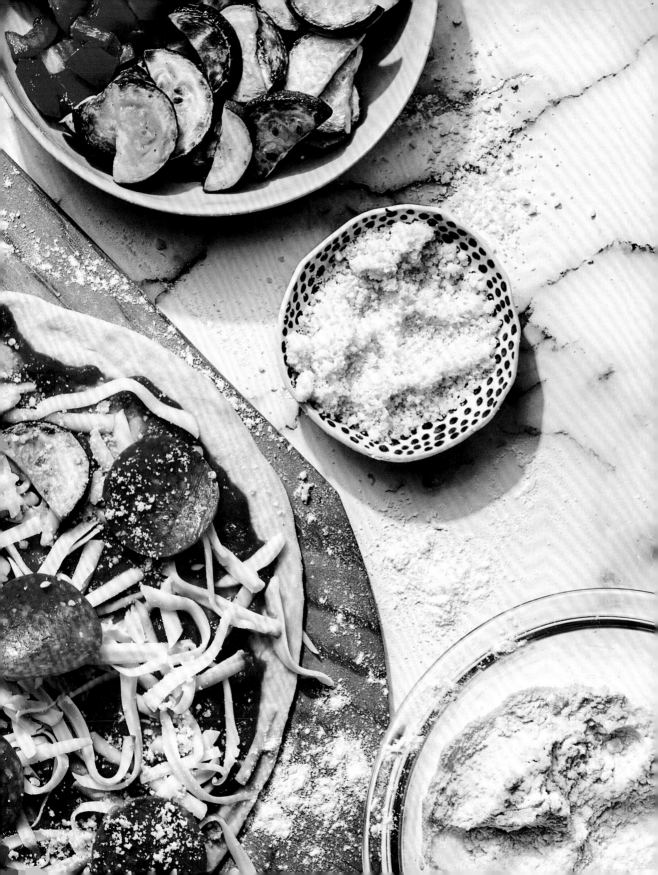

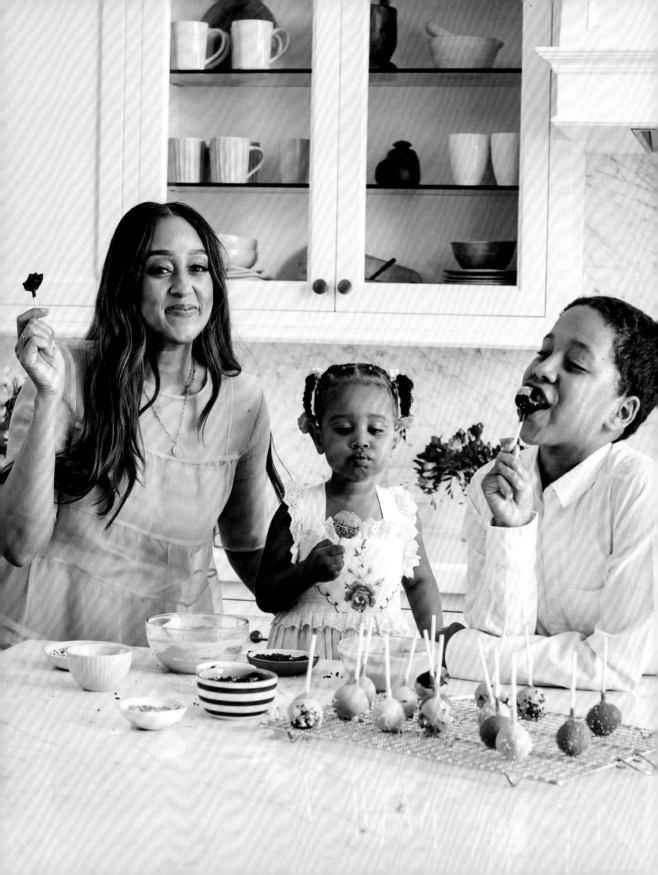

Sweets

Sweet Rolls

MAKES 15 ROLLS

PREP TIME: 20 minutes

TOTAL TIME: 1 hour 35 minutes
(includes rising time)

3¾ cups all-purpose flour,
   plus more for kneading

¼ cup sugar

2¼ teaspoons rapid-rise yeast

½ cup buttermilk
   (or the buttermilk swap;
   see page 73)

½ cup pineapple juice

5 tablespoons unsalted butter,
   melted

1½ teaspoons kosher salt

Nonstick cooking spray

2 tablespoons honey

Growing up, we always had Hawaiian rolls around the house for breakfast, lunch sandwiches, snacks, or dinner. While these might not be as sweet as those little bundles of joy, they are certainly as tempting! For this recipe, I use a zip-top bag instead of a bowl to mix and mingle the ingredients; it's easier and less of a mess. Hope you enjoy these as much as my family does!

In a 1-gallon zip-top plastic bag, combine 1 cup of the flour, the sugar, and yeast. Set aside.

In a glass measuring cup, combine the buttermilk and pineapple juice. Microwave until warm; the temperature should be 105° to 110°F. If you have a meat thermometer, you can use that to read the temperature, otherwise it should be hot but still touchable.

Pour the warm liquid into the bag of flour. Remove all the air from the bag and seal. Using clean hands, mix the ingredients inside by squishing everything together until you don't see any dry flour anymore. Let sit for 10 to 15 minutes. You should see bubbles in the bag.

Add another 1 cup of the flour, 3 tablespoons of the melted butter, and the salt to the bag. Remove all the air from the bag and mix again until you don't see any dry flour. Add 1¼ cups of the flour and continue mixing. Add another ¼ cup of the flour and mix. You want the mixture to come together; if it still looks wet, add another ¼ cup of flour and mix.

Tia's Tips

This recipe will also make a
9 × 5-inch loaf with a baking
time of 30 to 40 minutes, or until
the top is golden brown and
the bread springs back when you
touch it.

This recipe uses rapid-rise
(aka instant) yeast. Don't
substitute regular active dry
yeast in this recipe. Rapid-rise
yeast is a smaller particle, which
can be mixed into dry ingredients
instead of being combined
with water first to "bloom" and
rehydrate the yeast. I love how
scientific baking is; I still learn
something every day!

Lightly sprinkle some flour on a work surface. Dump
the dough onto the flour and knead until smooth, about
10 minutes. Add more flour, a little at a time, so the dough
doesn't stick to your work surface.

Spritz a small sheet pan or a 9 × 13-inch baking dish with
cooking spray. Divide the dough into 15 equal portions and
roll into balls. Place on the prepared pan or in the baking
dish about 1 inch apart, so they have some space when they
rise. Cover the pan or baking dish with a clean kitchen towel
and let sit in a warm place for 30 to 50 minutes.

Preheat the oven to 375°F.

In a small bowl, whisk together the remaining 2 tablespoons
melted butter and the honey until combined. Brush the top of
the rolls.

Bake until the tops of the rolls are golden brown, 20 to
25 minutes, rotating the pan front to back halfway through
baking. Serve warm.

Sweet Quick Bread Three Ways

SERVES 5 OR 6

PREP TIME: 15 minutes

TOTAL TIME: 1 hour 30 minutes

BASIC BATTER

Nonstick cooking spray

2½ cups all-purpose flour

2 teaspoons baking powder

1 teaspoon baking soda

½ teaspoon kosher salt

2 large eggs, at room temperature

1 cup buttermilk (or the buttermilk swap; see page 73)

⅓ cup canola oil

1 cup sugar

1 teaspoon pure vanilla extract

PUMPKIN-CHOCOLATE BREAD

1 tablespoon pumpkin pie spice

1 cup canned unsweetened pumpkin puree

1 cup semisweet chocolate chips

ZUCCHINI BREAD

2 cups grated zucchini

1 cup chopped walnuts

BANANA BREAD

3 ripe bananas, mashed

1 cup chopped pecans or chocolate chips

Who doesn't love a cozy loaf of pumpkin, banana, or zucchini bread? Sometimes, rather than (or in addition to) bringing a bottle of wine to a friend's house, I'll whip up one of these loaves as a gift instead with a note that reads: "Thanks for hosting us. I prepared your breakfast for tomorrow!" It's a cute little gesture that goes a long way.

Preheat the oven to 350°F. Spritz a 9 × 5-inch loaf pan with cooking spray.

PREPARE THE BASIC BATTER: In a large bowl, whisk together the flour, baking powder, baking soda, and salt until combined. In another bowl, whisk together the eggs, buttermilk, oil, sugar, and vanilla until combined. Add the wet ingredients to the dry and stir just until mixed.

CHOOSE YOUR BREAD VARIATION: Choose the variation you want, then use a rubber spatula to gently fold the pumpkin pie spice + pumpkin puree OR grated zucchini OR mashed bananas into the base batter until well combined. Try not to overmix. Gently fold in the chocolate chips or nuts until just mixed in. Scrape the batter into the prepared loaf pan.

Bake until a toothpick inserted in the center comes out clean, 55 to 65 minutes, rotating the pan front to back halfway through baking.

Let cool in the pan on a wire rack for 15 minutes, then turn out of the pan onto the rack to cool completely. Store in an airtight container at room temperature.

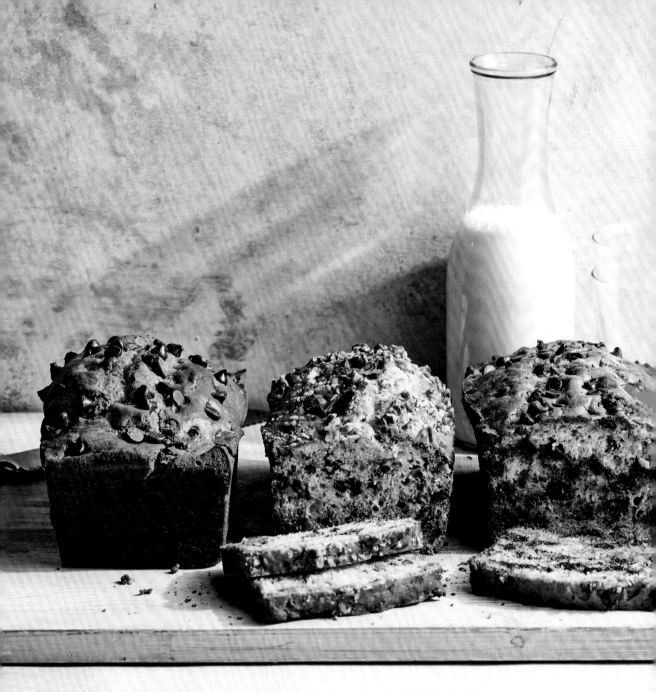

Tia's Tips

You can make these into muffins, too! Just adjust the cook time to 15 to 20 minutes, or until a toothpick inserted comes out clean.

Try not to overmix any batter that calls for flour. Overmixing releases the gluten in the flour and can make the bread dry and tough. If overmixed, let it sit for 15 to 30 minutes before baking. This will help relax the gluten a bit.

Frozen Yogurt Dots

SERVES 1

PREP TIME: 5 minutes

TOTAL TIME: at least 4 hours of freezing time

1 small container favorite yogurt

Kids really enjoy making *and* eating these buttons of frozen yogurt. Cree comes running in the door from school or playing outside asking for these treats when we have them. They're great by themselves in a bowl or on top of cereal.

If your yogurt has fruit on the bottom, give it a good stir to mix it up. Line a sheet pan with parchment or wax paper.

Place a 1-gallon zip-top plastic bag in a tall glass. Pull the outside edges of the bag over the edges of the glass and spoon the yogurt into the bag. Pick up the plastic bag and squeeze or push the yogurt to one corner of the bottom. Twist the top of the bag, while squeezing the air out. With scissors, snip off ¼ inch from the corner of the bag. Pipe a row of small dots (the size of a quarter or nickel) onto the lined baking sheet. As you pipe more dots, you'll get better with the size and shape.

Place in the freezer for at least 4 hours before eating. If you want to keep them longer, leave them on the baking sheet overnight, then transfer to an airtight container. They will keep in the freezer for at least 1 week.

Cookies in a Flash

MAKES 15 OR 16 COOKIES

PREP TIME: 10 minutes

TOTAL TIME: 20 minutes

1 large egg

1 cup hazelnut spread or cookie butter

¾ cup all-purpose flour

1 teaspoon baking powder

½ cup chocolate chips (optional)

Tia's Tips

Go crazy and add some flaky sea salt on top of the cookies before baking, if that is your thing.

Plain nut butter doesn't work here. It will be dry and tasteless.

Cookies made so easy! With only a few ingredients and one bowl, these tasty bites take less time to make than your traditional cookie and are an effortless recipe for the little ones. I use hazelnut spread or cookie butter because both have the fat and sugar needed for cookies, so you're not measuring out all that separately.

Preheat the oven to 350°F. Line two baking sheets with parchment paper.

In a large bowl, mix together the egg and hazelnut spread until fully combined. With a wooden spoon, stir in the flour and baking powder until combined. Stir in the chocolate chips, if using, but don't overmix. Using a small scoop, drop the mixture onto the lined baking sheets, setting them about 2 inches apart.

Bake for 4 minutes. Remove from the oven and use a spatula to gently push the cookies flat. Return to the oven and bake until the center of the cookie looks cooked, another 4 to 5 minutes. These cookies will be soft. Let cool on the baking sheets for a few minutes, then transfer to a wire rack to cool. Store in an airtight container for 5 to 7 days.

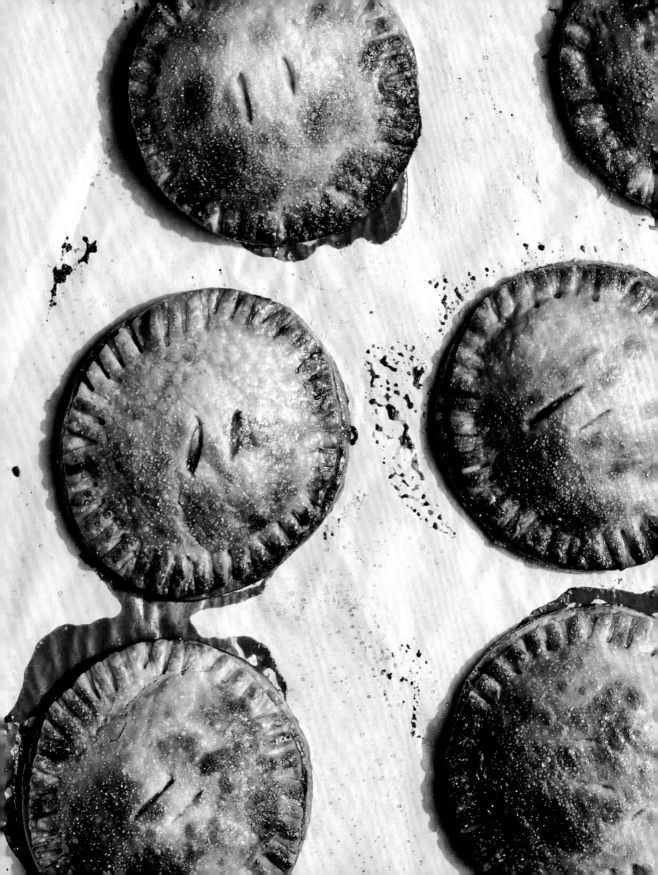

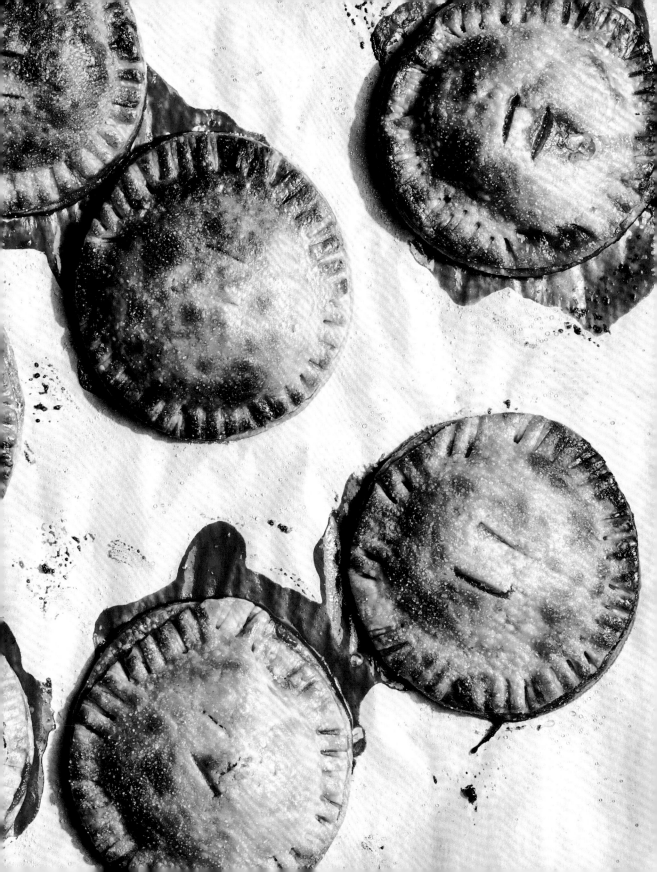

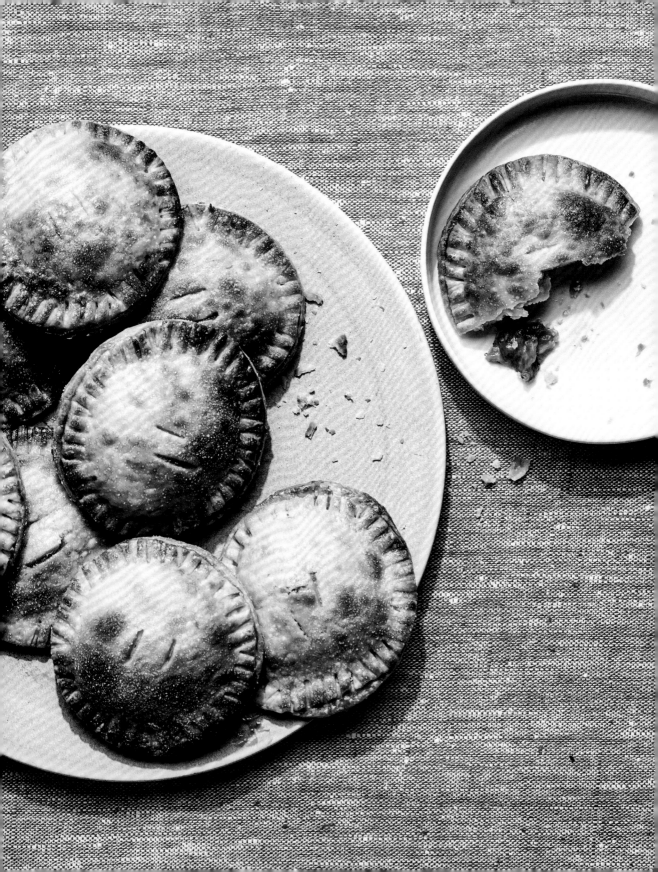

Strawberry Hand Pies

MAKES 12 PIES; SERVES 6 TO 8

PREP TIME: 15 minutes

TOTAL TIME: 30 minutes

2 store-bought pie crusts

All-purpose flour for dusting

6 strawberries, hulled and coarsely chopped

12 teaspoons jam of your choice

6 teaspoons cream cheese (optional)

1 large egg

Sugar, for sprinkling

Tia's Tips

Try blueberries, raspberries, or blackberries. And the cream cheese gives the center a rich creamy texture, but it's not necessary!

If you want to use apples or pears, you will need to sauté them first to soften them up before using as a filling.

Kids can make this entire treat all by themselves (but don't overstuff—the filling will ooze out)! Hint: Keep pie crust in your freezer at all times for quick sweet or savory yummies at a moment's notice.

Preheat the oven to 425°F. Line a baking sheet with parchment paper or a silicone baking mat.

Unroll the pie crust onto a lightly floured surface. Using a 3-inch round cutter, cut out as many rounds as possible. Gather up the scraps, roll into a ball, and roll out to ¼ inch thickness. Cut out more rounds. You should get about 12 rounds from each pie crust.

On the work surface, top half of the rounds with 1 tablespoon strawberries, 1 teaspoon jam, and ½ teaspoon cream cheese (if using), leaving a ½-inch border all around. In a small bowl, whisk the egg. Using clean fingertips, dip a finger into the egg wash and run it along the outer edge of the dough round. This acts like a glue to hold the top and bottom dough together.

Place another cut-out round of pie crust on top and use your fingertips to gently flatten out the dough to make a slightly thinner and larger dough round. This will help cover all the filling.

Using a fork, decoratively crimp the edges of the hand pie. With a sharp knife, cut a slit or two into the top crust. Brush with the egg wash and sprinkle with sugar. Place on the lined baking sheet.

Bake until golden brown, 15 to 20 minutes. Remove from the oven and let cool for 5 minutes before eating.

No-Bake Banana Cream Cake

SERVES 10 TO 12

PREP TIME: 30 minutes

TOTAL TIME: 8 hours 30 minutes
(includes chilling time)

2 (3.4-ounce) packages instant banana pudding or coconut cream pudding

4 cups cold whole milk or dairy-free creamer

1½ cups heavy cream

1 (14.4-ounce) box graham crackers

2 ripe bananas, thinly sliced

1 cup semisweet chocolate chips

I can't count how many times I've dipped my spoon into a banana cream pie, pudding, or cake. Kids love layering the graham crackers because they don't need to be perfect; they also love making the pudding because it's so easy!

Make the pudding according to the package directions, using cold milk (the cold makes it blend better).

In a large bowl, with an electric mixer, beat 1 cup of the heavy cream until stiff peaks form. With a rubber spatula, gently fold half of the whipped cream into the pudding—gentle strokes keep it light and fluffy; you don't want to deflate the mixture. Slowly fold in the remaining whipped cream until incorporated.

In a 9 × 13-inch baking dish, place graham crackers in a single layer, filling any holes by breaking them apart. Don't worry if they are overlapping slightly. Pour half of the vanilla pudding onto the graham crackers. Spread evenly and top with half the banana slices. Top with another layer of graham crackers, again breaking them apart if you need to fill in any open areas. Top with the remaining pudding and the remaining banana slices. Top with another layer of graham crackers. Place in the refrigerator uncovered until the ganache is made.

RECIPE CONTINUES

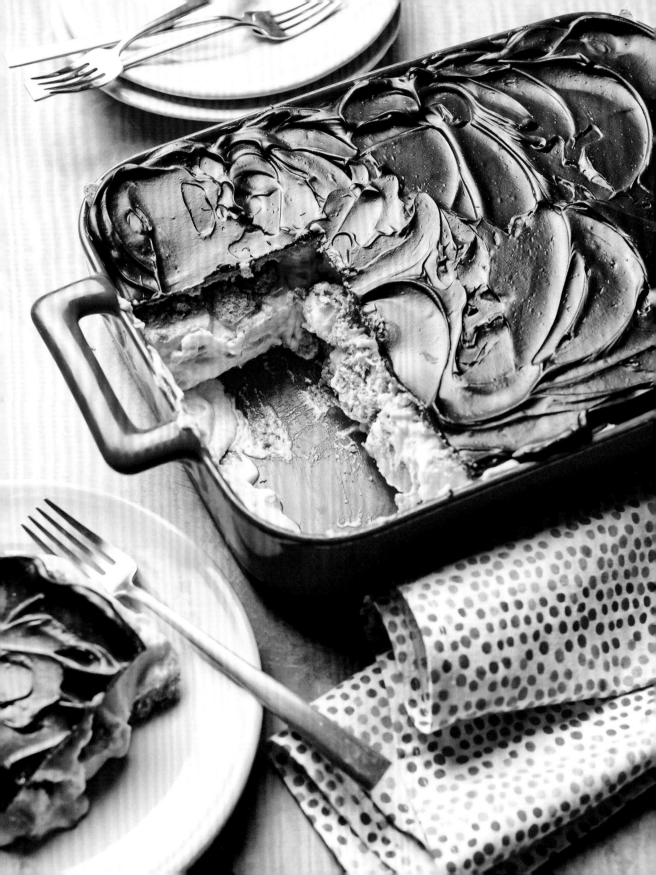

In a saucepan, heat the remaining ½ cup heavy cream over medium heat until hot but not boiling. Be careful not to boil and burn the cream, otherwise it will have a slightly burnt flavor. Remove from the heat. Add the chocolate chips and let sit for 1 minute. Gently and carefully whisk, until all the chocolate is melted and has a shiny, glossy look. Let sit until cooled but still pourable.

Pour the ganache over the cake and spread to cover the entire baking dish. Cover with plastic wrap tightly, so it does not touch the ganache. Refrigerate for at least 8 hours or overnight. The graham crackers will soften and become flavorful from the pudding. Cut into squares and serve. Holds great in the refrigerator for several days, too.

Tia's Tips

Graham crackers also come in chocolate flavor. Use those and switch up the pudding flavors with vanilla or white chocolate pudding. It's a win-win with any flavor.

This dessert is quick to make but does need some time in the refrigerator for the graham crackers to soften and absorb the flavors.

You could make this as individual servings in ramekins or small bowls.

No-Yeast Cinnamon Rolls

MAKES 12 ROLLS

PREP TIME: 30 minutes

TOTAL TIME: 1 hour

DOUGH

6 tablespoons unsalted butter,
    at room temperature

2¼ cups all-purpose flour,
    plus more for kneading

2 tablespoons granulated sugar

4 teaspoons baking powder

1 teaspoon kosher salt

¾ cup buttermilk
    (or the buttermilk swap;
    see page 73)

FILLING

½ cup packed light brown sugar

2 tablespoons unsalted butter,
    at room temperature

2 teaspoons ground cinnamon

¼ teaspoon kosher salt

ICING

1½ cups powdered sugar

1½ to 2 tablespoons whole milk

1 teaspoon pure vanilla extract

Don't let the lengthy instructions stop you from making these, because they are *a lot* easier to make than traditional cinnamon rolls, which require multiple risings and kneads and this and that. I give you pointers on how to work each step and what to do when things get sticky . . . *wink wink*, like the dough. Once you make these, I bet they'll become a Sunday-morning staple.

Preheat the oven to 325°F. Grease a 9 × 13-inch baking dish with 1 tablespoon soft butter. Set aside.

MAKE THE DOUGH: In a large bowl, whisk together the flour, granulated sugar, baking powder, and salt. Using clean hands, add the remaining 5 tablespoons butter to the flour mixture and mix so it becomes crumbly. Add the buttermilk and stir with a rubber spatula until a dough is formed. This will be sticky and wet. Sprinkle with a tablespoon of flour and dump onto a floured work surface. Sprinkle the work surface with another tablespoon of flour and form the dough into a disc. What we are trying to do here is make the dough come together without stickiness by adding small amounts of flour at a time. This will keep the dough flaky and moist.

Once you have a disc of dough, return it to the bowl and chill for at least 30 minutes in the refrigerator or in the freezer for 15 minutes. You want the butter to get cold again. (At this point, the dough can be kept in the refrigerator for a few days or the freezer for 3 months.)

RECIPE CONTINUES

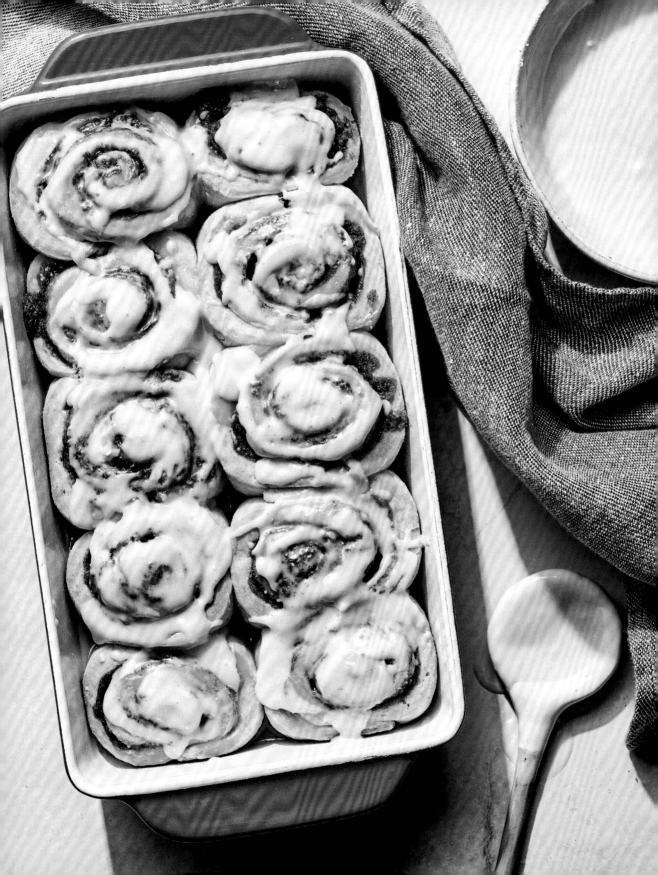

Tia's Tip

Let's talk fillings! Use the base filling recipe and channel your sense of adventure. Add ¼ cup chopped nuts, ⅓ cup chocolate chips, ⅓ cup shredded coconut, ½ cup sautéed apples, or ½ cup crispy bacon. Let your imagination run free!

WHILE THE DOUGH IS CHILLING, MAKE THE FILLING: In a medium bowl, combine the brown sugar, butter, cinnamon, and salt. The mixture will be slightly crumbly. Set aside.

Remove the dough from the refrigerator and dust a work surface with flour. Roll out to a 10 × 13-inch rectangle. When rolling the dough, move it around and lightly dust the surface with flour. This will help keep it from sticking. Sprinkle the filling evenly over the dough, leaving a 1-inch border around the edges.

Starting at a long side, carefully roll into a log. If the log seems soft, place on a tray and refrigerate until firm.

You are going to cut this into 12 pieces. To do so, start by cutting the log in the middle and then cut both of those pieces in half. Now you have 4 equal sections. Cut each of those 4 sections into 3 pieces. Place the rounds cut-side up in the prepared baking dish about 1 inch apart.

Bake until the edges are slightly browned, 30 to 35 minutes.

WHILE THE ROLLS ARE BAKING, MAKE THE ICING: In a small bowl, stir together the powdered sugar, 1½ tablespoons milk, and the vanilla. The icing should be pourable. If you need to add more milk, do so 1 teaspoon at a time. If it becomes too liquid-y, add more powdered sugar.

Remove the rolls from the oven and let sit for 5 minutes. While warm, drizzle with icing and serve from the baking dish.

Individual Chocolate Chip Cookie

SERVES 1

PREP TIME: 3 minutes

TOTAL TIME: 4 minutes

2 tablespoons light brown sugar

1 tablespoon salted butter, melted

2 teaspoons whole or 2% milk

3 tablespoons all-purpose flour
  or 1-to-1 gluten-free flour

⅛ teaspoon baking soda

1 tablespoon chocolate chips,
  semisweet, milk, or dark

1 tablespoon chopped nuts
  (optional)

Sometimes I crave a sweet treat at night, but do *not* crave the work of a whole batch of cookies. In those dire times, I make one cookie. And when I'm feeling extra sweet, I top it with ice cream and am over the moon in 4 minutes! Kids can make this without the worry of oven ouchies, but let them know the plate will be hot to the touch when leaving the microwave!

In a large bowl, stir together the brown sugar, melted butter, and milk. Add the flour and baking soda and stir just until fully mixed. Stir in the chocolate chips and nuts (if using). The mixture will be loose, but you can fill an ice cream scoop with the cookie mixture. Scoop onto a microwave-safe plate and flatten to ½ inch thick. Microwave for 1 minute at full power. Let sit for a minute or two before eating.

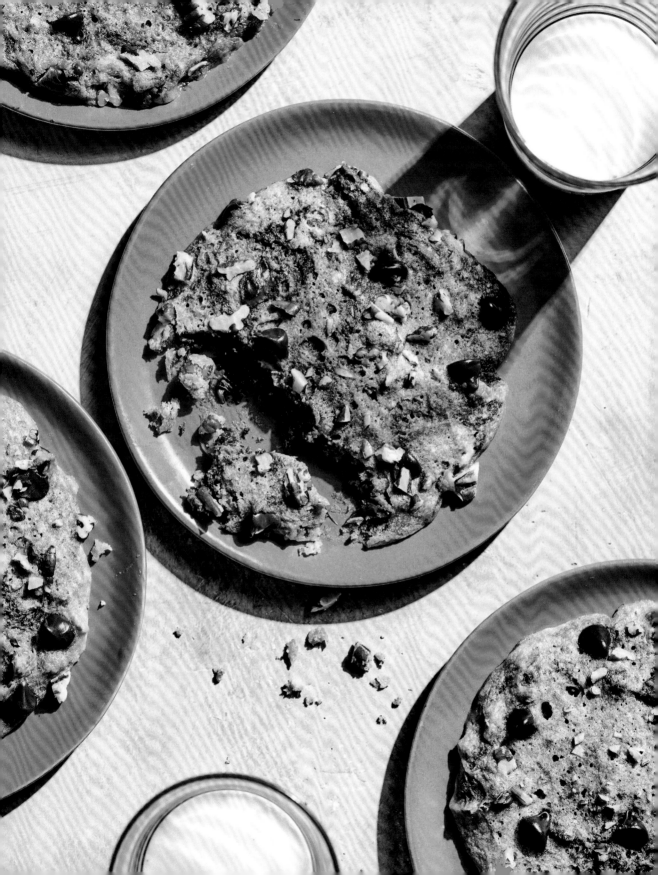

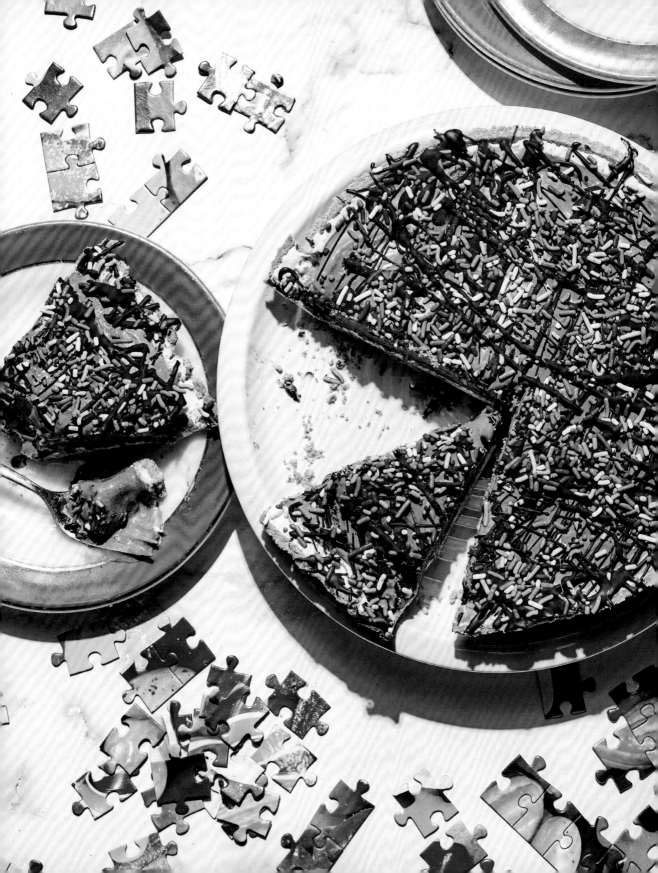

Frozen S'mores Pie

SERVES 8

PREP TIME: 30 minutes

TOTAL TIME: 8 hours or overnight

1 gallon favorite ice cream

1 cup marshmallow creme

1 store-bought graham cracker pie crust

CHOCOLATE HARD SHELL TOPPING

¾ cup dark chocolate chips

1 tablespoon coconut oil

Tia's Tips

You can add sprinkles, chopped cookies, and nuts to the top of the pie, but you will have to work fast before the chocolate hardens. This is great to do with the kids; you can drizzle while they sprinkle.

Add a surprise layer of fudge on the crust before adding the ice cream if you're looking for a fudgier treat. You can also use two different flavors of ice cream to form layers.

And feel free to top with whipped cream, or anything you feel will warm the souls of the eaters!

You can customize this scrumptious dessert for that special someone by using their favorite ice cream and toppings. This recipe teaches you the basic technique for an ice cream pie that will have them (whoever they are) asking for s'more!

Let the ice cream sit at room temperature for 20 to 30 minutes. You want this ice cream soft and spreadable.

Meanwhile, spread a thin layer of marshmallow creme over the entire graham cracker crust. Place in the freezer for 10 minutes, while your ice cream is getting soft.

Remove the crust from the freezer and spoon the ice cream into the crust. Push down into the crust to fill in any open spaces. Spread until even, while mounding in the middle. Place in the freezer for 8 hours or overnight.

MAKE THE CHOCOLATE HARD SHELL TOPPING:
In a small microwave-safe bowl, combine the dark chocolate and coconut oil and microwave for 45 seconds. Remove and stir; if the chocolate is still chunky, return to the microwave for 30 seconds. Remove and stir until melted. Allow the melted chocolate to cool slightly, not until hard but until the bowl is no longer hot. This will stop the ice cream from melting while topping with chocolate.

Remove the ice cream pie from the freezer. Starting in the center, pour the chocolate over the pie. Work quickly, allowing the chocolate to drizzle down the pie and harden. Save about ¼ cup chocolate. Drizzle the reserved chocolate back and forth over the hardened chocolate to create a design. Serve immediately.

Banana Pops

SERVES 4

PREP TIME: 15 minutes

TOTAL TIME: 25 minutes

4 bananas

CHOCOLATE DIP

4 tablespoons coconut oil, melted and warm

2 tablespoons honey, agave, or maple syrup

3 tablespoons unsweetened cacao powder

¼ teaspoon sea salt

TOPPINGS

Sprinkles

Crushed graham crackers

Chopped chocolate

Drizzled melted white chocolate

Chopped nuts

Tia's Tips

These bananas can be eaten right after the chocolate sets or the next day when they are frozen all the way through.

Bananas freeze well and stay creamy, but if you leave a frozen banana at room temperature too long it will turn mushy. So serve straight from the freezer.

I remember going to Disneyland and rushing straight to the ice cream vendors for a frozen banana. My goodness, those were a highlight of my day at the park! Turns out they're super easy to make at home and fun for the kids, too.

Peel the bananas and cut in half crosswise. Push a wooden ice pop stick into the cut side of the banana, about halfway in. Arrange on a parchment-lined baking sheet. Place in the freezer for 10 minutes.

MEANWHILE, MAKE THE CHOCOLATE DIP: In a glass measuring cup, whisk together the coconut oil, honey, cacao powder, and salt until smooth. The oil should be warm enough to melt the honey and make it smooth.

ASSEMBLE THE POPS: Remove the bananas from the freezer. Holding a banana by the wooden stick, dip it into the chocolate sauce. Swirl to coat the banana and return to the baking sheet. Working fast, sprinkle your chosen toppings onto the banana as soon as you set it down. The chocolate will harden quickly. Once you are done dipping all the bananas, return to the freezer for 15 minutes.

Keep any leftover bananas in the freezer; they'll be good for 2 weeks.

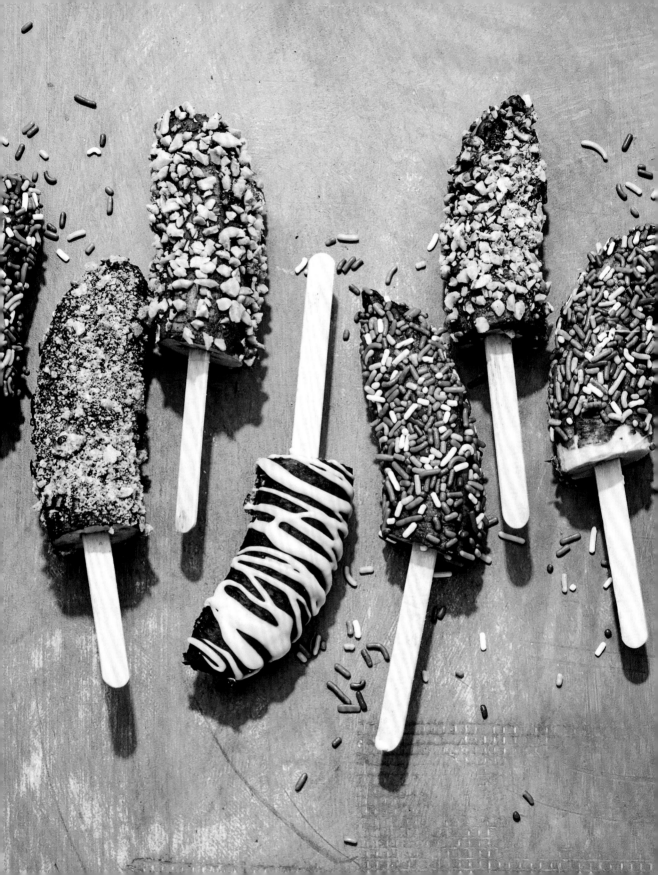

Easy-Peasy Confetti Cake

with Buttercream Frosting

SERVES 6 TO 8

PREP TIME: 20 minutes

TOTAL TIME: 1 hour 45 minutes

Nonstick cooking spray

2 cups all-purpose flour

1 (3.4-ounce) box instant vanilla pudding mix

2 teaspoons baking powder

1 teaspoon kosher salt

¾ cup (1½ sticks) unsalted butter, at room temperature

1¼ cups granulated sugar

4 large eggs, at room temperature

1 tablespoon pure vanilla extract

½ cup milk, at room temperature

¼ cup rainbow sprinkles

BUTTERCREAM FROSTING

1½ cups (3 sticks) unsalted butter, at room temperature

1 teaspoon pure vanilla extract

½ teaspoon kosher salt

4½ cups powdered sugar

Milk (if necessary)

Rainbow sprinkles

This cake is a playful, creative way to decorate a cake and build that massive slice of our dreams. Decorate it as you like, and know that this is a simple, reliable alternative to the cake mix you can buy at the store.

Preheat the oven to 350°F. Spritz a 9-inch round cake pan with cooking spray. To make doubly sure the cake comes out of the pan, cut a 9-inch round of parchment paper and add to the bottom of the pan, then spritz the paper.

In a large bowl, whisk together the flour, pudding mix, baking powder, and salt. Set aside.

In a separate large bowl, with an electric mixer, cream the butter and granulated sugar until the color is light and the mixture is fluffy, 3 to 5 minutes. Add the eggs one at a time, making sure the egg is fully incorporated before you add another one. Mix in the vanilla.

Add the flour mixture to the butter mixture in three additions, alternating with the milk, beginning and ending with the flour. Mix well each time you add the ingredients, but don't overmix. Use a rubber spatula to gently fold the sprinkles into the batter, taking extra care not to overmix or the sprinkles will bleed all their color and you will have streaks of color instead of sprinkles of color.

Pour the batter into the prepared pan and level the top. Bake until a toothpick inserted into the center of the cake comes out clean, 50 to 60 minutes, rotating the pan front to back halfway through.

Tia's Tip

This cake has a moist and dense center. Try it as a chocolate cake by adding ½ cup cacao powder to the dry ingredients and use chocolate pudding instead of the vanilla. You can even swap the vanilla extract for chocolate extract, but it's not necessary.

Let the cake cool in the pan for at least 10 to 15 minutes, then turn out of the pan onto a rack to cool completely before frosting. Remove the parchment paper round from the bottom of the cake.

MAKE THE BUTTERCREAM FROSTING: In a large bowl, with an electric mixer, cream the butter until smooth. Beat in the vanilla and salt. Add the powdered sugar 1 cup at a time, beating until incorporated. When all the sugar is added, if the frosting is too stiff, add milk 1 tablespoon at a time, until the frosting looks creamy.

Set the cooled cake right-side up on a cutting board and use a serrated knife to cut off the top of the cake. You want this to be flat and level. Place the cake on a plate or tray that can go into the freezer. Frost the top of the cake with a thick layer of frosting, about 1 inch. Level the frosting so it is smooth. Place the cake in the freezer for 30 minutes. Remove from the freezer and cut the cake into quarters. You are trying to make 4 even wedges.

Place a cake wedge frosting-side up on a serving platter. Stack the rest of the wedges on top, frosting-side up (you are making what looks like a giant wedge of cake). Try to get them as straight and lined up as possible. If you have long skewers, push 1 or 2 down into the center of the cake to support it. Frost the top and outsides of the cake, but do not frost any part that shows the layered inside of the cake. Decorate with more sprinkles on the frosting and serve. If the frosting has gotten too soft, place the cake in the refrigerator to firm up.

There you have it, the biggest slice of cake you ever did see.

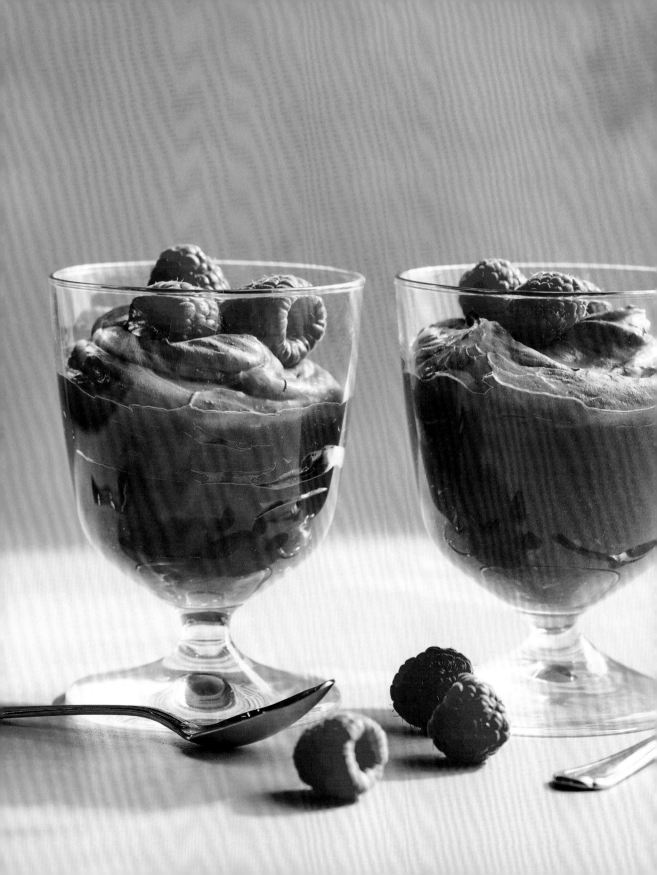

Dairy-Free Creamy Chocolate Pudding

SERVES 4 OR 5

PREP TIME: 15 minutes

TOTAL TIME: 12 hours 15 minutes (includes chilling time)

2 (13.5-ounce) cans full-fat coconut milk or cream, refrigerated for at least 12 hours

½ cup unsweetened cacao powder

¼ cup powdered sugar, sifted

½ teaspoon mint extract (optional)

Once you've tried this, you won't believe it's dairy free! It's creamy, chocolaty, silky, and everything you want when imagining a luscious spoonful of chocolate. If you take the time to chill it, it's as creamy as gelato.

Scoop out the thick coconut cream from the cans of coconut milk and add to a mixing bowl. Reserve the remaining coconut liquid for cooking or smoothies.

With a stand mixer or hand mixer, whip the coconut cream until creamy, 3 to 4 minutes. It will also become thicker and almost double in size, like whipped cream. Add the cacao powder, sugar, and mint extract (if using). Whip until fully incorporated.

Serve right away or transfer to a large serving bowl, cover, and refrigerate until ready to serve.

Tia's Tip

Top with raspberries or strawberries during the summer. Sprinkle with crushed cookies and peppermint candies for the holidays, and you'll be transported to the North Pole!

Cookie Cake Balls

MAKES 48 CAKE BALLS

PREP TIME: 30 minutes

TOTAL TIME: 1 hour 45 minutes
(includes chilling time)

40 cream-filled chocolate
sandwich cookies

1 (8-ounce) package cream
cheese, at room temperature

1 (12-ounce) bag semisweet
or dark chocolate chips

TOPPINGS

Sprinkles

Drizzled melted white chocolate

Crushed peppermints

Crushed pretzels

Mini chocolate, white chocolate,
or butterscotch chips

Sometimes the easiest desserts make the biggest splash.
These are all store-bought items and make a super-fun
activity for the kids. Depending on the occasion, you can
spruce them up however you please! For the holidays,
crush some of those candy canes you have lying around;
at Halloween cut chocolate wafer cookies in half and
make them into bat wings; for birthdays, coat them with
celebratory rainbow sprinkles; or keep them as is for an
extravagant Tuesday.

In a food processor, pulse the cookies until finely chopped.
Add the cream cheese and blend until combined. With a
small ice cream scoop, scoop the mixture into 1-inch balls
and roll with clean hands. Set on a tray and refrigerate for
15 minutes to firm up.

In a 2-cup glass measuring cup, fill halfway with chocolate
chips. Microwave for 45 seconds, remove, and stir. Return
to the microwave and heat for 30 seconds, remove, and stir.
The heat of the chocolate and the glass cup will melt any
unmelted chocolate, just keep stirring. If there are still chunks,
place in the microwave for another 20 seconds.

Line a baking sheet with parchment or wax paper. Using
2 forks, dip the cookie balls in the melted chocolate. Let
the excess chocolate drip back into the cup. Place on the
lined baking sheet. While the chocolate is still wet, add any
toppings.

Refrigerate for 1 hour to firm up. Store in the refrigerator for
3 to 5 days.

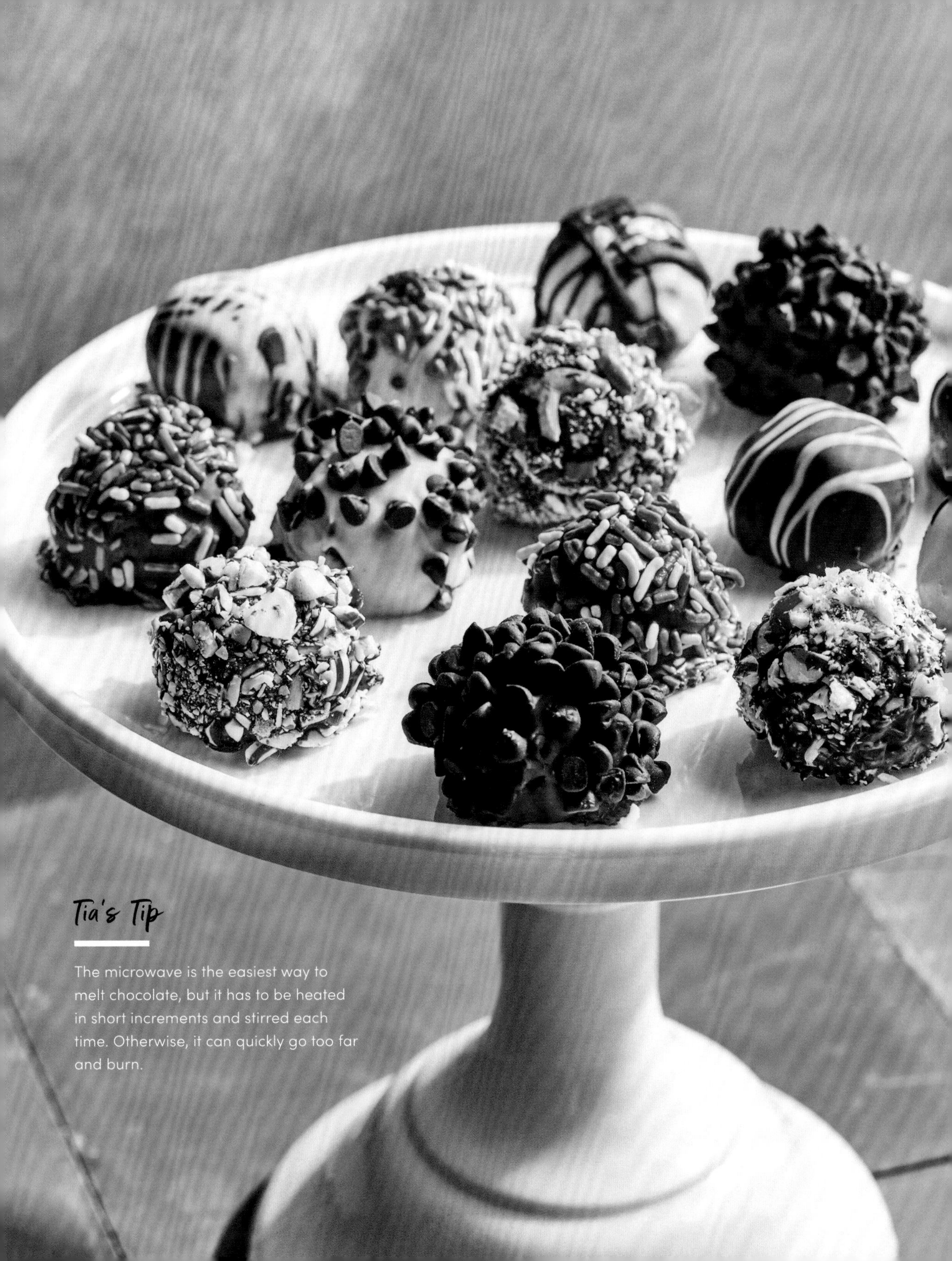

Tia's Tip

The microwave is the easiest way to melt chocolate, but it has to be heated in short increments and stirred each time. Otherwise, it can quickly go too far and burn.

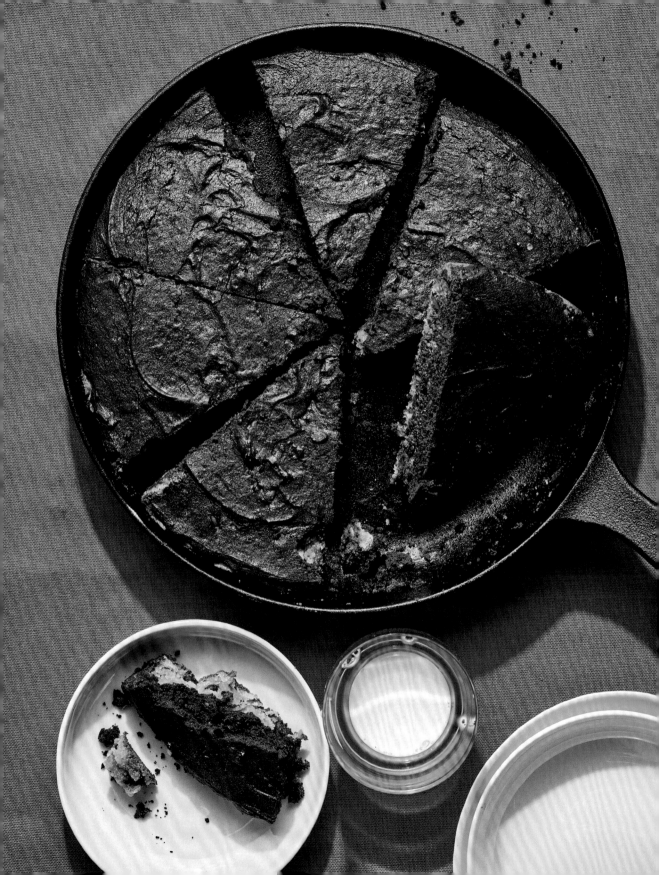

Brookies

MAKES 12 TO 16 BARS

PREP TIME: 15 minutes

TOTAL TIME: 35 minutes, plus cooling time

COOKIE LAYER

Nonstick cooking spray

½ cup (1 stick) unsalted butter, melted

½ cup packed light brown sugar

¼ cup granulated sugar

½ teaspoon pure vanilla extract

1 large egg

1¼ cups all-purpose flour

½ teaspoon kosher salt

1 cup semisweet chocolate chips

BROWNIE LAYER

½ cup granulated sugar

½ cup (1 stick) unsalted butter, melted

1 teaspoon pure vanilla extract

2 large eggs

½ cup unsweetened cacao powder

½ cup all-purpose flour

¼ teaspoon baking powder

½ teaspoon kosher salt

For when you can't choose between the cookies or a brownie on the dessert line, this is the best of both worlds! Cree can make this recipe from start to finish (with me swooping in to help for the oven part, of course).
Two bowls, anticipation of brownies and cookies in one bite, and just a little elbow grease are all it takes.

Preheat the oven to 350°F. Line a 9 × 13-inch baking dish with parchment or foil so it overhangs the two long edges. Lightly spritz with cooking spray.

MAKE THE COOKIE LAYER: In a large bowl, whisk together the melted butter, brown sugar, granulated sugar, and vanilla until fully combined. Add the egg and whisk until the batter looks light and creamy. Stir in the flour and salt and mix until just combined. Stir in the chocolate chips, until just incorporated. Dollop into the prepared pan and spread out evenly. Set aside.

MAKE THE BROWNIE LAYER: In another large bowl, whisk together the granulated sugar, melted butter, and vanilla. Add the eggs and beat well. Whisk in the cacao powder until well combined. Using a rubber spatula, stir in the flour, baking powder, and salt until combined. Pour the brownie batter over the cookie layer. Gently spread evenly in the pan.

Bake until a toothpick inserted in the center comes out clean, 20 to 25 minutes, rotating the pan front to back halfway through cooking. Let cool completely, then cut into 12 to 16 bars.

Baked Cinnamon Sugar Donuts

MAKES 12 TO 13 DONUTS OR 24 MINI DONUT HOLES

PREP TIME: 20 minutes

TOTAL TIME: 35 minutes

Nonstick cooking spray

1 cup sugar, plus more for the pan(s)

1¼ cups whole or 2% milk

1 teaspoon apple cider vinegar or distilled white vinegar

2 cups all-purpose flour

2 teaspoons baking powder

1 teaspoon ground cinnamon

½ teaspoon kosher salt

1 large egg

2 tablespoons unsalted butter, melted

2 teaspoons pure vanilla extract

TOPPING

½ cup sugar

1 teaspoon ground cinnamon

If your loved ones weren't satisfied by the apple "donuts" earlier in the book, then go for the real deal. Well, kind of. These are baked not fried!

Preheat the oven to 350°F. Spritz either two 6-hole donut pans or a 24-hole mini muffin pan with cooking spray. Sprinkle with sugar. Turn the pan upside down over the sink and tap out any extra sugar. This helps prevent the donuts from sticking.

In a medium bowl, stir together the milk and vinegar. Let sit for 10 minutes.

In a large bowl, whisk together the flour, 1 cup sugar, baking powder, cinnamon, and salt. To the milk and vinegar bowl, whisk in the egg, melted butter, and vanilla. Stir the wet mixture into the dry ingredients until just combined. Do not overmix!

Spoon the batter into the pan(s), filling each hole three-quarters full. Do not overfill or they will overflow while baking.

Transfer to the oven and bake until a toothpick inserted in the thickest part of a donut hole or donut comes out clean, 10 to 12 minutes for the mini muffin pan and 15 to 17 minutes for the donut pans. Note that the donuts do not turn a golden brown; instead they will remain a very pale color. Let cool for 5 minutes before topping.

MEANWHILE, MAKE THE TOPPING: In a small bowl, whisk together the sugar and cinnamon. One at a time, gently remove a warm donut and add to the bowl of cinnamon sugar. Sprinkle with the sugar and place on a platter.

Store in an airtight container for 1 week.

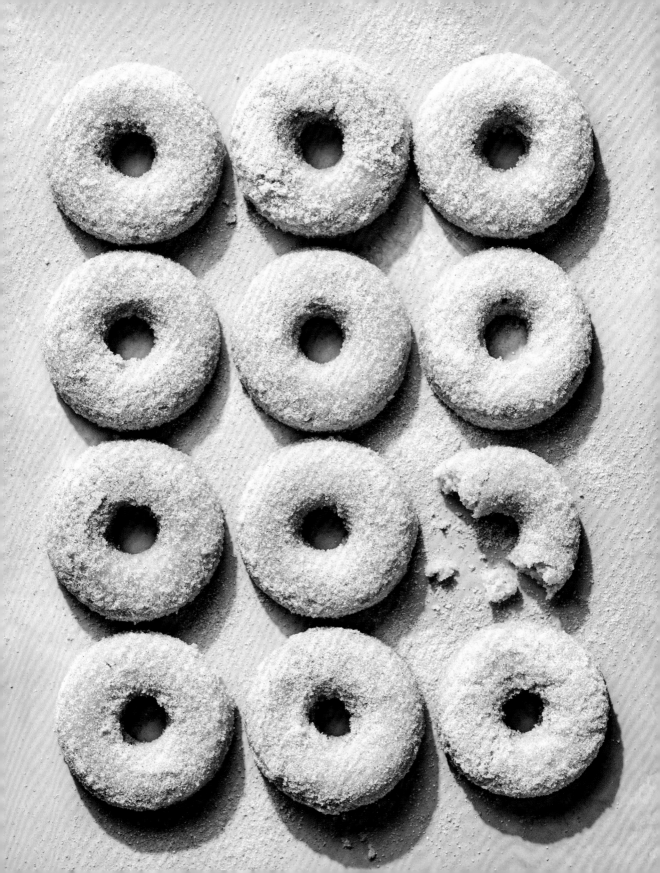

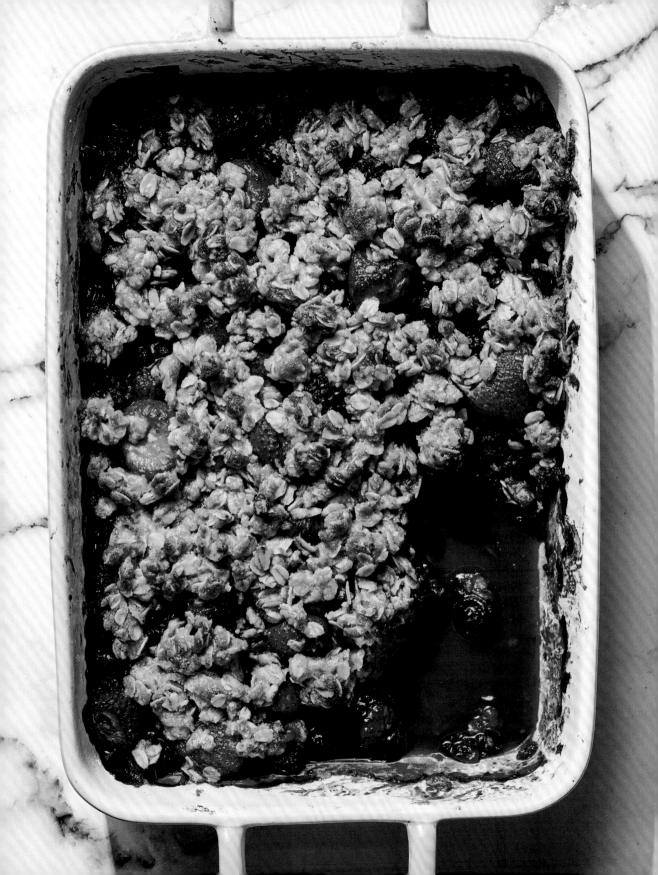

Any Fruit Crisp

SERVES 6 TO 8

PREP TIME: 10 minutes

TOTAL TIME: 40 minutes

1 tablespoon unsalted butter

7 cups cut-up fruit of choice, frozen and/or fresh

2 tablespoons sugar

2 tablespoons cornstarch

½ teaspoon kosher salt

TOPPING

1 cup old-fashioned rolled oats

½ cup all-purpose flour

½ cup packed light brown sugar

½ cup (1 stick) unsalted butter, melted

FOR SERVING

Whipped cream

Ice cream

Fruit crisps seem a lot more difficult than they really are. It's a bit of tossing together with a bit of baking, with no extra bother. And this recipe, again, allows you to do whatever you want with it!

Preheat the oven to 425°F. Using the unsalted butter, lightly grease a 10-inch ovenproof skillet or 9 × 13-inch baking dish.

Pile the fruit into the skillet or dish. Sprinkle it with the sugar, cornstarch, and salt. Gently toss until the cornstarch is mixed in. Set aside.

MAKE THE TOPPING: In a medium bowl, stir together the oats, flour, and brown sugar. Pour in the melted butter and stir until fully combined and crumbly. Pour over the fruit, trying to cover most of it.

Bake until the crisp topping gets golden brown and the fruit starts to bubble, 30 to 35 minutes.

TO SERVE: Let sit for 10 minutes before serving. Serve with whipped cream or ice cream.

Tia's Tips

Any type of fruit will work for this amazing crisp. If using apples, pears, or peaches, peel and thinly slice. Use fruit that is in season, as it will be sweeter.

You could also make a bunch of individual servings in ramekins with everyone's favorite fruit.

RESOURCES

Balanced Kitchen

Michael Eisenstein, "The Hunt for a Healthy Microbiome," *Nature* (January 2020): doi:https://doi.org/10.1038/d41586-020-00193-3

How to Decipher Egg Carton Labels (n.d.). Retrieved from The Humane Society of the United States: https://www.humanesociety.org/resources/how-decipher-egg-carton-labels

Meat, Poultry, and Fish: Picking Healthy Proteins. (2017, March 26). Retrieved from American Heart Association: https://www.heart.org/en/healthy-living/healthy-eating/eat-smart/nutrition-basics/meat-poultry-and-fish-picking-healthy-proteins

Eco-Certified Seafood (n.d.). Retrieved from Monterey Bay Aquarium Seafood Watch: https://www.seafoodwatch.org/seafood-recommendations/eco-certification

Whole Grains 101. (n.d.). Retrieved from Old Ways Whole Grains Council: https://wholegrainscouncil.org/whole-grains-101

Reese Oxner, "For Subway, A Ruling Not So Sweet. Irish Court Says Its Bread Isn't Bread" NPR (October 2020): https://www.npr.org/2020/10/01/919189045/for-subway-a-ruling-not-so-sweet-irish-court-says-its-bread-isnt-bread

How Much Sugar Do You Eat? You May Be Surprised! (n.d.). Retrieved from New Hampshire Department of Health and Human Services: https://www.dhhs.nh.gov/dphs/nhp/documents/sugar.pdf

Seasonal Produce Guide. (n.d.). Retrieved from SNAP-Ed Connection U.S. Department of Agriculture: https://snaped.fns.usda.gov/seasonal-produce-guide

(n.d.). *What's on Your Plate?* Retrieved from MyPlate, U.S. Department of Agriculture: https://www.myplate.gov

Staff writer, "The Secrets of the Caribbean Cuisine," *WPB Magazine* (August 2015): https://www.wpbmagazine.com/secrets-of-the-caribbean-cuisine

Andrew Dorenburg and Karen A. Page, *The Flavor Bible: The Essential Guide to Culinary Creativity, Based on the Wisdom of America's Most Imaginative Chefs* (New York: Little, Brown & Co., 2008).

Recipe Substitutions. (n.d.). Retrieved from Dartmouth University: https://www.dartmouth.edu/~patl/substitutions.shtml

Giuseppe Di Palma, M. B., "Italy: Agriculture, Forestry, and Fishing," *Encyclopædia Britannica:* (October 2020) https://www.britannica.com/place/Italy/Agriculture-forestry-and-fishing#ref26991

History of Spanish Food. (n.d.). Retrieved from Enforex: https://www.enforex.com/culture/history-spanish-food.html

Prepared Kitchen

How to Store Fruits and Veggies. (n.d.). Retrieved from Fruits & Veggies Half Your Plate: https://www.halfyourplate.ca/fruits -and-veggies/store-fruits-veggies

Safe Minimum Cooking Temperatures Charts. (Date Last Reviewed April 12, 2019). Retrieved from FoodSafety.gov: https:// www.foodsafety.gov/food-safety-charts /safe-minimum-cooking-temperature

Kid's Kitchen

Cooking with Kids: A Guide to Kitchen Tasks for Every Age. (2020, July 30). Retrieved from Taste of Home: https://www.tasteof home.com/article/cooking-with-kids-a -guide-to-kitchen-tasks-for-every-age

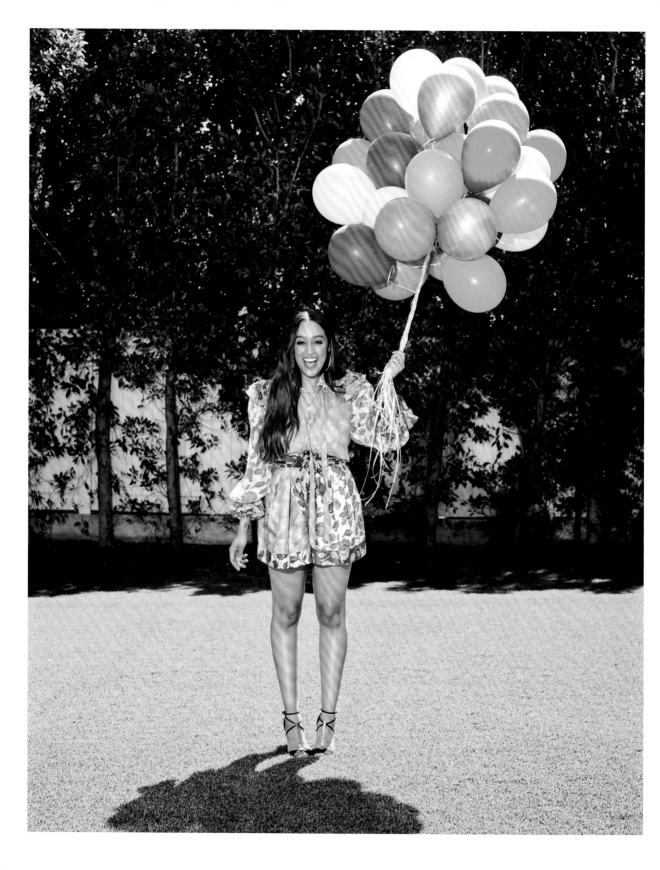

ACKNOWLEDGMENTS

We all know it takes a village to take on a project like this, and I couldn't do this without my incredible team. Thank you to my smart and savvy manager, Adam Griffin, at Vault Entertainment; my relentless and creative project manager, Ryan Bundra; my forward-thinking publicist, Cece Yorke, and everyone at True PR; my knowledgeable and meticulous attorneys, Fred Toczek and Jordan Rojas; my wise book agent at UTA, Brandi Bowles; and all of my friends who have been with me every chop, dice, simmer, and sauté along the way. Also, I would like to send a very special thanks to my collaborators, Danielle Bernabe and Angela Gaines: I could not have done this without all of your incredible work.

And finally, I want to thank everyone who has picked up this book and decided to have FUN in the kitchen. Trust me when I say it's an inspirational and life-changing place to be. I'm so proud of you! You've just taken a big step toward your better health and expanding your good taste. You've got this!

INDEX

ABOUT THE AUTHOR

TIA MOWRY-HARDRICT is an actress, producer, author, lifestyle influencer, and business owner. Tia has been in the public eye for twenty-five years; she first came on the scene with her hit comedy series *Sister, Sister* and currently stars in the Netflix series *Family Reunion.*

Tia, in partnership with Kin Community, created the YouTube channel "Tia Mowry's Quick Fix." The go-to online resource provides weekly uploads to help viewers solve life's little dilemmas quickly. It also stands as the company's fastest growing channel to date, garnering more than 2 million followers.

Tia invited fans into her kitchen with the release of her first cookbook—the bestseller *Whole New You*, by Ballantine Books. She also wrote the book *Oh, Baby! Pregnancy Tales and Advice from One Hot Mama to Another*, which quickly became a national bestseller, delivering the lowdown in a frank, hilarious guide to modern pregnancy.

In 2020, Tia launched Anser supplements in partnership with BioSchwartz, debuting a line of simple, high-quality, and affordable products that inspire people of all backgrounds to take charge of their own health.